T0226511

Patient Safety

Guest Editor

DONNA S. WATSON, RN, MSN, CNOR, ARNP-BC

PERIOPERATIVE NURSING CLINICS

www.periopnursing.theclinics.com

Consulting Editor
NANCY GIRARD, PhD, RN, FAAN

December 2008 • Volume 3 • Number 4

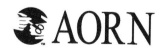

SAUNDERS an imprint of ELSEVIER, Inc.

W.B. SAUNDERS COMPANY
A Division of Elsevier Inc.

1600 John F. Kennedy Boulevard • Suite 1800 • Philadelphia, Pennsylvania 19103-2899

http://www.periopnursing.theclinics.com

PERIOPERATIVE NURSING CLINICS Volume 3, Number 4
December 2008 ISSN 1556-7931, ISBN-13: 978-1-4160-6336-0, ISBN-10: 1-4160-6336-6

Editor: Katie Hartner
Developmental Editor: Theresa Collier

Perioperative Nursing Clinics (ISSN 1556-7931) is published quarterly by Elsevier, 360 ParkAvenue South, New York, NY 10010. Months of issue are March, June, September and December. Business and Editorial Offices: 1600 John F. Kennedy Blvd., Suite 1800, Philadelphia, PA 19103-2899. Customer Service Office: 11830 Westline Industrial Drive, St. Louis, MO 63146. Periodicals postage paid at New York, NY and at additional mailing offices. Subscription prices are $116.00 per year (domestic individuals), $209.00 per year (domestic institutions), $58.00 per year (domestic students/residents), $116.00 per year (Canadian individuals), $240.00 per year (Canadian institutions), $150 per year (international individuals), $240 per year (international institutions), and $62.00 per year (International and Canadian students/residents). Foreign air speed delivery is included in all Clinics subscription prices. All prices are subject to change without notice. **POSTMASTER:** Send change of address to *Perioperative Nursing Clinics*, Customer Service (orders, claims, online, change of address): Elsevier Periodicals Customer Service, 11830 Westline Industrial Drive, St. Louis, MO 63146. Tel: 1-800-654-2452 (U.S. and Canada). Fax: 314-523-5170. E-mail: journalscustomerservice-usa@elsevier.com (for print support); journalsonlinesupport-usa@elsevier.com (for online support).

Reprints. For copies of 100 or more, of articles in this publication, please contact the Commercial Reprints Department, Elsevier Inc., 360 Park Avenue South, New York, NY 10010-1710. Tel. (212) 633-3812; Fax: (212) 462-1935; email: reprints@elsevier.com.

Printed and bound by CPI Group (UK) Ltd, Croydon, CR0 4YY

Transferred to Digital Print 2011

Contributors

CONSULTING EDITOR

NANCY GIRARD, PhD, RN, FAAN
Consultant, Boerne, Texas

GUEST EDITOR

DONNA S. WATSON, RN, MSN, CNOR, ARNP-BC
Senior Clinical Educator, Covidien
Energy-Based Devices, Boulder,
Colorado

AUTHORS

JENNIFER S. BARNETT, RN, MSN, ARNP
Cascade Vascular Associates, Tacoma,
Washington

SANDRA C. BIBB, DNSc, RN
Associate Professor and Chair, Department
of Health Systems, Risk and Contingency
Management, Uniformed Services University
of the Health Sciences, Graduate School of
Nursing, Bethesda, Maryland

LINDA BRAZEN, RN, MSN, CNOR
Clinical Nurse Specialist/Educator, University
of Colorado Hospital, Denver, Colorado

SANDY BROWN, RN
Coordinator, Transfusion-Free Medicine and
Surgery Program, Franciscan Health System,
St. Joseph Medical Center, Tacoma,
Washington

LISA COLE, MAJ, MSN, RN, CNOR
Perioperative Clinical Nurse Specialist and
Element Leader of Surgical Support Services,
96th Medical Group, Eglin USAF Regional
Hospital, Eglin Air Force Base, Florida

ALECIA COOPER, RN, MBA, CNOR
Senior Vice President, Clinical and Marketing
Services, Medline Industries, Inc., Mundelein,
Illinois

LINDA J. DECARLO, RN, MSN, MBA, CNOR, RNFA, ARNP
Cascade Vascular Associates, Tacoma,
Washington

VIVIAN M. DEVINE, PCNS, CNOR, RN
United States Navy; Formerly, Graduate
Student (2004–2006), Uniformed Services
University of the Health Sciences, Bethesda,
Maryland

CLAIRE R. EVERSON, RN, CNOR, CCAP
PeriOperative/Endoscopy Clinical Educator,
Banner Desert Medical Center, Mesa, Arizona

JARRELL FOX, Program Manager,
Transfusion-Free Medicine and Surgery
Program, Franciscan Health System,
St. Joseph Medical Center, Tacoma,
Washington

ALLAN FRANKEL, MD
Faculty, Division of General Medicine, Brigham
and Women's Hospital; Instructor, Harvard
Medical School; Faculty, Institute for
Healthcare Improvement, Boston,
Massachusetts

JILL GARRETT, RN, CPHQ
Perioperative Care Manager, Memorial Health
System, Colorado Springs, Colorado

BRADLEE GOECKNER, LCDR, MSN, RN, CNOR
Clinical Coordinator, Perioperative Department, Naval Medical Center San Diego, San Diego, California

RODNEY W. HICKS, PhD, MSN, MPA, FNP-BC, FAANP
UMC Endowed Chair for Patient Safety and Professor, Anita Thigpen Perry School of Nursing, Texas Tech University Health Sciences Center, Lubbock, Texas

AILEEN KILLEN, PhD, RN
Patient Safety Program Director, Memorial Sloan Kettering Cancer Center, New York, New York

CECIL A. KING, MS, RN, CNOR
Clinical Educator, Perioperative Services, Cape Cod Hospital, Hyannis, Massachusetts

MICHAEL LEONARD, MD
National Physician Leader for Patient Safety, and Kaiser Permanente Faculty, Institute for Healthcare Improvement, Boston, Massachusetts

SHARON A. MCNAMARA, RN, MS, CNOR
Director of Surgical Services, WakeMed Health and Hospitals, Raleigh, North Carolina

JAN ODOM-FORREN, MS, RN, CPAN, FAAN
Perianesthesia Nursing Consultant, Louisville; Instructor, University of Kentucky, Lexington, Kentucky

CHRISTOPHER R. SMITH, LCDR, NC, USN, MSN, MHR, CNOR
Perioperative Clinical Nurse Specialist, Main Operating Room, National Naval Medical Center, Bethesda, Maryland

REBECCA VIGIL, RN
Coordinator, Transfusion-Free Medicine and Surgery Program, Franciscan Health System, St. Joseph Medical Center, Tacoma, Washington

CHASITY BURROWS WALTERS, MSN, RN
Patient Safety Facilitator, Memorial Sloan Kettering Cancer Center, New York, New York

LINDA J. WANZER, Col (Ret), MSN, RN, CNOR
Director, Perioperative Clinical Nurse Specialist Program; and Assistant Professor of Nursing, Graduate School of Nursing, Uniformed Services University of the Health Sciences, Bethesda, Maryland

Contents

Operating room safety is dependent on professional and regulatory requirements that mandate skill levels, documentation standards, monitoring, and equipment. Protocols exist for almost every procedure performed, and overall there is excellent management. Physicians, nurses, and technicians rely on these characteristics to support delivery of safe care. Most practitioners have had the experience of working in suboptimal operating room conditions. There are many causes for this state, including mechanisms for reimbursement that impede alignment of interests between physicians and hospitals; limited interdisciplinary training; and perceptions about the roles of personnel that have not kept pace with the changing nature of care delivery.

As one of the most complex health care environments, the operating room is fraught with weaknesses and practices in need of process improvements. To make the operating room a safer environment for patients, a systems perspective is necessary. To provide a basis for readers, fundamentals of human factors, ergonomics, and systems thinking are discussed. Various strategies and resources are provided to assist readers with the design of a safer operating room. This information is presented in consideration of the varying availability of resources within institutions, allowing for allocation of efforts where possible to balance the operating room as a system.

Patient safety initiatives at the national and local level, launched by public and private stakeholders, and embracing large goals or small steps, have proved to be remarkably effective in improving patient safety, reducing medical errors, and saving money. Such initiatives may begin with sweeping concerns, but they ultimately boil down to a list of tactics. Many of these tactical steps are simple, inexpensive, and not particularly difficult to implement. It is highly encouraging that the solutions to many knotty and seemingly overwhelming health care problems can actually be found in a series of small, specific steps crafted in the form of specific health care initiatives.

for prospective population health research and program development for the perioperative continuum.

Claire R. Everson

The potential for a fire during surgical, perioperative, and interventional procedures should always be recognized. Free-standing ambulatory surgery centers, endoscopy centers, imaging centers, and physician's offices have gaps in emergency services and response teams. These areas need well-understood plans, intense orientation, and ongoing education because there is no one else to rely on until the fire department arrives. This article discusses fire safety issues, including prevention, suppression, evacuation, and communication, and highlights current regulations for patient safety issues.

Jarrell Fox, Sandy Brown, and Rebecca Vigil

The risks and benefits of a request for nonblood medical or surgical management must be weighed against a patient's constitutional right to refuse treatment. Thorough assessment, planning, and preparation optimize a patient's status to undergo surgery without transfusions. Thoughtful selection of surgical approach, meticulous hemostasis, and blood salvage with reinfusion can minimize blood loss. Continuous patient assessment, supportive measures, and selective phlebotomy allow safe recovery. An educated, organized, and well-equipped team can manage the medical and surgical care without the use of blood transfusions; not only do we have the tools but also the ethical responsibility to do so.

Jan Odom-Forren

The use of sedation administered by nonanesthesia providers has increased exponentially over the past decade. Moderate sedation is safe but has potential adverse reactions such as hypoxemia, apnea, hypotension, airway obstruction, and cardiopulmonary arrest. Patient safety is the responsibility of every person on the perioperative team and relies on an effective sedation delivery system to keep the patient from harm. Performing safe and effective sedation involves several aspects of sedation, including the persons administering the sedation, the educational processes involved, the environment in which the sedation is conducted, patient-specific information processes, and guidelines and protocols of the institution. Future areas of research in clinical studies include safety and efficacy studies, applications of new technology, and procedural sedation and analgesia adjuncts.

Jennifer S. Barnett and Linda J. DeCarlo

Deep venous thrombosis and pulmonary embolism are significant safety issues for surgical patients. Types of surgery and individual patient risk factors affect the probability of developing thromboembolic events. Nurses are in a strategic position to impact patient safety and help reduce health care expenditures by collaborating with the surgical team in implementing appropriate deep venous thrombosis prophylaxis

Perioperative Nursing Clinics

THE CLINICS ARE NOW AVAILABLE ONLINE!

Access your subscription at:
www.theclinics.com

Foreword

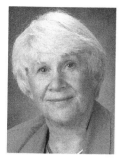

Nancy Girard, PhD, RN, FAAN
Consulting Editor

I am pleased to present this issue of *Perioperative Nursing Clinics* to you, our valued reader. Donna Watson, a respected perioperative leader, is the guest editor for this issue titled "Patient Safety", and she has compiled an impressive list of authors and topics. As you read this issue, I hope it will trigger new thoughts that you can apply to your working environment, and also that it will update your knowledge and interest in those practices with which you are familiar. Safety in patient care is highlighted extensively these days, but this concern has always been the backbone of perioperative nursing. With the national spotlight on problems with safety in surgical care and examples of tragic and preventable outcomes, there are now accepted team and institutional concerns. Safety in patient care is a topic that will continue to be a concern in perioperative care. It is not a problem that, once solved, will go away. Thus, this issue is of vital importance to the reader, and hopefully it will ultimately benefit each and every patient undergoing surgery.

As the new Consulting Editor, I hope to continue the tradition begun in 2006. The previous consulting editor was Patricia C. Seiffert, who is an outstanding perioperative leader. With her efforts, *Perioperative Nursing Clinics* premiered in March 2006 with the issue titled "Bariatric Surgery," and the series continued to grow through the next two years. My heartiest thanks go to Patricia Seiffert for developing this fine *Clinics*.

Many of you are familiar with my past work. I served as editor of *Seminars* in *Perioperative Nursing*, a Saunders journal published for many years. Then I moved to the AORN Journal as Editor-in-Chief for several years. These editorial experiences were invaluable. I am very pleased to be back with Elsevier and to serve as the new Consulting Editor for *Perioperative Nursing Clinics*. I promise to work diligently to present you with up-to-date information that will be useful and educational in the clinical area.

The series will continue to be offered quarterly, focusing on one topic per issue. There will continue to be an outstanding Guest Editor per issue; one that is an expert in his or her field. We have planned some exciting topics in the coming year, such as leadership, education, and research topics, presented in a way that should appeal to the reader and be applicable to clinical practice. We will continue to collaborate with The Association of periOperative Registered Nurses (AORN) and will tie in sources, resources, guidelines, and standards of practice as defined by the organization for select articles. We also will identify national and federal standards and guidelines, many of which you will see in articles in this issue.

I would love to hear from you and learn what topics you would like to see in the future. If you would be interested in serving as guest editor or would like to write an article for one of the planned future issues, please do not hesitate to contact me.

Nancy Girard, PhD, RN, FAAN
Consultant
8910 Buckskin Drive
Boerne, TX 78006-5565, USA

E-mail address:
ngirard2@satx.rr.com (N. Girard)

Perioperative Nursing Clinics 3 (2008) xi
doi:10.1016/j.cpen.2008.09.001

periopnursing.theclinics.com

Preface

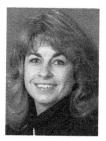

Donna S. Watson, RN, MSN, CNOR, ARNP-BC
Guest Editor

The process of improving patient safety issues to prevent patient harm is complex and challenging. The philosophical foundation for nursing care is based on the fundamental principle of patient safety, but with the current complex health care environment, it continues to require the necessity to be addressed with every patient encounter. The Institute of Medicine's publicized report forever changed business as usual when it revealed that approximately 44,000–98,000 deaths directly related to preventable medical errors occur annually.[1] Medical errors would rank as the sixth leading cause of death in the United States if medical errors were included as a ranking in the leading cause of death. Thus, deaths attributed to medical errors would surpass annual deaths caused by Alzheimer's disease, diabetes mellitus, influenza and pneumonia, nephritis, nephritic syndrome, nephritis or septicemia.[2] Death is considered preventable, and there lies the challenge; thus do no harm.

Practice in the surgical services area is a dynamic environment requiring staff to interface constantly with challenges related to environment, equipment, systems, and personality. On a daily basis, professional nurses and surgical teams deal with these ambiguous entities, which require flexibility and precise decision making that will guide the surgical patient through an uneventful safe perioperative course. This does not occur without planning, commitment, competency, and expertise.

Preventing medical errors in the perioperative environment requires continued diligence toward the end goal. This issue of *Perioperative Nursing Clinics* contains a series of articles from experts on a variety of patient safety topics, which will assist perioperative team members who may struggle with complex patient safety issues. The authors provide a comprehensive analysis of the key national Patient Safety Initiatives, proactively impacting patient safety and specifically patient safety in the surgical services setting, to help the reader better understand and define patient safety. This issue addresses some of the problems with creating a just culture and provides a recommendation for successful implementation. Competency development, as it relates to patient safety, is addressed in an easy-to-understand format. Additionally, the issue would not be complete without addressing some of the high risk patient safety issues in the surgical services area, including the prevention of deep venous thrombosis, bloodless surgery, surgical counts, retained foreign objects, wrong site surgery, wrong patient, wrong procedure, fire safety, safe administration of moderate sedation, and medication errors.

It has been my pleasure to work with experts across the country to share practical solutions to some patient safety issues.

Each article provides valuable information that is practical and easy to implement. Patient safety is an individual, team, and facility commitment. One preventable error is one too many.

Donna S. Watson, RN, MSN, CNOR, ARNP-BC
Covidien Energy-Based Devices
5920 Longbow Drive
Boulder, CO 80301-3299, USA

E-mail address:
watsoncnor@comcast.net (D.S. Watson)

REFERENCES

1. Institute of Medicine. To err is human: building a safer health system. Washington, DC: National Academy Press; 2000. p. 1.
2. Heron MP, Hoyert DL, Xu J, et al. Deaths: preliminary data for 2006. National Vital Statistics Reports 2008;56(16):5 (June 11, 2008). Available at: http://www.cdc.gov/hchs/nvss.htm. Accessed August 14, 2008.

Perioperative Nursing Clinics 3 (2008) xiii
doi:10.1016/j.cpen.2008.08.013

Essential Components for a Patient Safety Strategy

Allan Frankel, MD[a,b,c,*], Michael Leonard, MD[c]

KEYWORDS

- Patient saftey • Teamwork • Leadership • Innovation
- Cultural measurement • Reliable care • Reliability

The safety of operating rooms is dependent in large measure on the professional and regulatory requirements that mandate skill levels, documentation standards, appropriate monitoring, and well-maintained equipment. Prescriptive and detailed protocols exist for almost every procedure performed, and although variation based on surgical and anesthesia preference is allowed, overall there is excellent management of the technical aspects. Experienced operating room physicians, nurses, and technicians come to rely on these operating room characteristics to support the delivery of safe care. Most practitioners, however, at some time—and some much of the time—have had the experience of working in suboptimal operating room conditions because the level of procedural complexity in even the simplest of operative procedures is not matched by the necessary team coordination, leadership engagement, or departmental perspective that encompasses all the prerequisites for reliable delivery of care. There are many causes for this current state that include, depending on country, the mechanisms for reimbursement that impede alignment of interests between physicians and hospitals;[1] the limited interdisciplinary training of the various disciplines—surgery, anesthesia, nursing, and technician—that promote hierarchy and undervalue core team characteristics; and historical perceptions about the roles of physicians, nurses, and ancillary personnel that have not kept pace with the changing nature of care delivery.[2]

As far back as 1909, Ernest Avery Codman, a Boston orthopedic surgeon, openly challenged the then current orthodoxy and proposed that Boston hospitals and physicians publicly share their clinical outcomes, complications, and harm. Wisely, he resigned his hospital position shortly before going public with this request, so he could not be thrown off the staff. Despite that, criticisms of him were severe. One hundred years later, his wishes are being realized across the United States at a rapidly accelerating pace.[3] The 1991 Harvard Medical Practice Study that evaluated errors in 30 hospitals in New York State and that ultimately led to the now highly quoted number of 98,000 unnecessary deaths per year—accruing from health care error—has forced the industry to reflect on the apparent contradiction that the edifices built to care for patients are harming many of them.[4,5] From these reflections a science of comprehensive patient safety has been woven from the threads of disciplines such as engineering, cognitive psychology, and sociology. Combined with the quickening pace of electronic health record deployment, the movement toward demonstrable quality and value in medical care is happening quickly.

THE CASE FOR SAFE AND RELIABLE HEALTH CARE

The 1991 Harvard Medical Practice Study was the seminal article leading to the 1999 Institute of Medicine (IOM) report, *To Err is Human*,[6] and that report has led to great public and business

[a] Division of General Medicine, Brigham and Women's Hospital, Boston, MA, USA
[b] Harvard Medical School, Boston, MA, USA
[c] Institute for Healthcare Improvement, Boston, MA, USA
* Corresponding author. 15 White Tail Lane, Sudbury, MA 01776.
E-mail address: allan.frankel@lotusforum.com (A. Frankel).

Perioperative Nursing Clinics 3 (2008) 263–276
doi:10.1016/j.cpen.2008.08.004

awareness of quality and safety problems in the health care industry. The media have fueled the public's interest and businesses have formed advocacy groups, such as Leapfrog,[7] to focus attention on this critical topic. The American government program, Medicare, with approximately $600 billion in annual spending, recently announced it would not pay for care resulting from medical errors.[8] Large private insurers are quickly following suit. Aetna just announced it will not pay for care related to the "28 never events" defined by the National Quality Forum.[9]

Rapidly developing transparency in the market about safety and quality will be a major driver. Beth Israel Deaconess Hospital in Boston now posts its quality measures on their Web site, including their recent Joint Commission accreditation survey.[10] New York City Health and Hospitals Corporation, the largest public care system in the United States, has committed to following suit. The State of Minnesota publicly posts on the Internet all their hospital's reported never events, such as wrong site surgeries and retained foreign objects during surgery.[11] Several other states are quickly following suit. Geisinger Clinic in Pennsylvania now offers a warranty on heart surgery,[12] in which specified complications are cared for without charge. Given the impressive care processes they have developed, this is a logical way to message their superior care and compete in the market. The successful hospitals and health systems in this new rapidly transparent market will be the ones that apply systematic solutions to enhance patient safety. Other bright spots in the systematic approaches taken by large care systems include Kaiser Permanente and Ascension Health in the areas of surgical and obstetric safety, and through Institute for Healthcare Improvement (IHI) initiatives, such as the 100,000 Lives Campaign and the 5 Million Lives Campaign.[13]

There has been a great deal of activity to improve the safety and quality of care since the IOM report. Currently there are pockets of excellence, but broadly there is much more work to do and fundamental gaps in the quality and safety of health care as it exists today. Well-intentioned projects and efforts to improve patient safety have met with variable results. Overall, however, in the absence of systematic, solutions-based approaches, health care organizations are unlikely to achieve sustained excellence in clinical safety and quality. This article describes the authors' current thinking as to the necessary elements for a comprehensive program to help insure safe and reliable care for every patient every day. The surgical environment is an obvious one to which these programs should be applied and surgical nursing will play a huge role in shaping the efforts. They also will shape, in turn, nursing.

THE OPERATING ROOM AS A SYSTEM

To begin, think of safety from an engineering perspective, which considers how safe a system is based on how reliably it produces its product or, restated, based on the frequency of its defects. Engineers think about

- The reliability of achieving the desired outcome not just once but repeatedly
- Evaluating the processes leading to the desired outcome
- Analyzing in detail the indivisible steps that, together, make up the process

In operating rooms, the process has dozens and in some cases hundreds of sequential steps. The reliability of each of the steps—that is, whether or not each step occurs as it should—determines whether or not the desired outcome will be achieved.

Ultimately, system safety and reliability are determined by the rate of defects in each step. When defect rates are multiplied, it becomes increasingly likely that they lead to an undesired outcome. The result could, but not always, be of clinical harm to patients. Patients may be fine, but the process nevertheless may have significant flaws that predispose patients to a greater than reasonable risk of harm. This is an indication that although a current patient did not suffer an adverse event, the next patient might not be so lucky.

If the clinical perspective is combined with the engineer's, a reliable operative procedure will see patients safely through because all of the steps in the processes have reliably small and known defect rates.

PROCESS STEPS

Taking this theoretic construct and making it real, consider that each step in the process is an individual and indivisible action, as when, for example, an operating room gets a patient's chart. The simple act of holding the chart in one's hands is a step in the process of evaluating a patient before beginning a surgical procedure.

Once a chart is in hand, there are a series of other steps that might include checking the hematocrit box in the laboratory section, checking the consent box in the front of the chart, and perusing the blood pressure and heart rate trends in the clinical section. These three steps (or four if blood pressure and heart rate are on different pages of the clinical section) depend on several processes of their own, such as a secretary or assistant placing the chart in a convenient location and checking the correct information in the correct place in the chart. The process steps undertaken each have failure rates of their own and determine whether or not the information is present in the chart when it reaches the nurse.

Suffice it to say that any operative procedure performed in any location, viewed from this perspective, is made up of dozens to hundreds or thousands of steps, and every one of them has an intrinsic defect rate; some might be single steps but many also will have associated processes that determine their defect rate.

To the degree that each step's defect rates can be quantified, the safety of a system is measurable, and the measure is not only whether or not the outcome is achieved but also whether or not the processes may be replicated over and over again. To a large extent, safety is a system property determined by a system's reliability.

ACHIEVING RELIABILITY IN SYSTEMS

Operating rooms have done a remarkably good job of making themselves reliable and safe, albeit in a health care industry that has been slow to incorporate many key features of reliable systems.[14] The Harvard anesthesia practice standards[15] generated in the 1980s and adopted across the United States are a shining example of standardization of anesthesia care that has helped improve the safety of the specialty. These standards identified minimum monitoring expectations now commonly used in every surgical procedure. They affect all of surgical nursing and influenced the broad adoption of pulse oximetry and capnography.

Another rich source of reliability in operating rooms has in the past derived from promoting the interoperability of its practitioners. Although one anesthesia provider or nurse may begin a procedure, it has been likely that many other members in a department would be capable of replacing them and might be called on to do so. This continues to be likely in many departments in which transfers of care occur daily; however, the limitations in interoperability are growing as equipment and surgical specialties become more specialized and require increasingly sophisticated knowledge of technique and machinery. The implications of increased specialization and technical complexity inevitably will influence decisions about caseload and case type regarding timing of cases, after-hours procedures, and, in all likelihood, credentialing of all operating room practitioners.

Reliability is feasible only when a group of interdependent factors are effectively woven together to produce a whole cloth.[16] The threads are the key; their individual quality determines the appearance, and potentially the beauty, of the final tapestry. There are six types of threads in the weave. They are:

- An environment of continuous learning
- A just and fair culture[17,18]
- An environment of enthusiasm for teamwork
- Leaders engaged in safety and reliability through the use of data[19,20]
- Effective flow of information
- Intelligent engagement of patients in their own care

Weaving occurs only through concerted effort at multiple levels, starting with a goal, that takes precedence over all others, to achieve reliability. Organizations and departments that do embark on the road to greater reliability find that the end result positively influences patient care and employee satisfaction;[21] it is obvious even to outside observers. To some extent this applies to all operating room practitioners as they arrive in a location to participate in a procedure. The initial reaction, that gut feeling about the quality of relationships, and the safety of the environment should be taken seriously, for it is likely to be a good barometer of the risk inherent in the environment.[8]

AN ENVIRONMENT OF CONTINUOUS LEARNING

The paradigm of a learning environment is Toyota Industries. They lead the auto industry in size and sales, and the enthusiasm of their car owners is well known. Toyota employees make suggestions for improving the work they do an average of 46 times per year and do so with the knowledge that a significant number of their suggestions will be tested and, if found worthy, adopted and spread. This process of applying the insights of the frontline workers to change and improvement applies not only to the production of their cars but also to the fundamental work of improvement itself. Toyota strives not only to continuously improve their car production but also to improve the way they "do improvement."[22] In other words, if a change in a procedure takes 1 month today, Toyota would be seeking ideas so that a year from now it could perform that change in 3 weeks. If Toyota daily receives 10 useful suggestions from a department, then 1 year from now their goal would be to receive 12 or 15. Their perspective is that improvement is always feasible and there is always waste to be removed from their processes.

The fact that in a prior quarter wasted effort and materials decreased as a result of focused improvement efforts is immaterial. There is, unrelentingly, always more to be achieved.[23,24]

Where is health care in this picture and how does the example of Toyota apply to anesthesiologists when they arrive in a remote location to give an anesthetic? Physicians and hospitals have, for decades, had a guild relationship in which single physicians plied their trade within the walls of a hospital but with singularly insular perspectives. In the past 20 years a different health care industry has begun to emerge, built on a flood of hard evidence from randomized controlled clinical trials. Groups of clinicians are now providing service-line delivery across the spectrum of care-associated specific diseases.[12]

An environment of continuous learning in health care requires the presence of certain structural elements and the ability to execute ideas. The most basic of structural elements is the meeting of the clinical, unit-based leadership to consider information about unreliable events and decide on actions to remedy them.[25] Surgical procedures will take place safely only in those clinical units whose leaders are able to orchestrate this process, and nursing must, to repeat, must be an integral part of the leadership discussions in that unit. Multidisciplinary staff should meet on a regular basis to examine the straightforward operational issues in units, from items as specific as getting drugs to the right places in each room to the flow of patients through the entire suite.

The information collected at such meetings should be collated and evaluated so that remedies to any problems, potential problems, or concerns may be pursued. As in Toyota and other industries with reputations for high reliability,[26] listening to the front line and acting on their concerns is a key to ensuring a safe process. This requires an environment or culture that makes it easy to bring problems to light and a teamwork structure that supports this process. Both of these can be evaluated.

A JUST AND FAIR CULTURE

A just and fair culture in health care is one in which individuals fully appreciate that although they are accountable for their actions, they will not be held accountable for system flaws.[17,27] This culture provides a framework for looking at errors and adverse events to quickly and consistently determine whether or not an individual nurse or physician involved in the event is problematic at a behavioral or technical skill level or whether or not he or she was set to fail by system flaw. This means evaluating the culpability of an individual after an error, accident, or adverse event by using a simple algorithm that asks (1) Did the individual mean to cause harm? (2) Did the individual come to work impaired (by drugs, alcohol, and so forth)? (3) Did the individual follow reasonable rules that others who have similar knowledge and skills would have followed? and (4) Did the individual have a history of participating in or causing unsafe acts?[27] If the answers are, respectively, no, no, yes, and no, then there is no personal blame accrued. The full appreciation of this means the organization believes, and that belief is corroborated by the actions of the organization, that there exists a reasonable mechanism to evaluate untoward events, regardless of the outcome of the event. Implicit in this, and an extension of it, is that actions are evaluated based on what is best for patients and not on who is supporting the actions. Hierarchy, formal or informal, is not material in discussions of this sort.

When evaluating medication errors, the majority of the time the algorithm identifies capable conscientious individuals working in an unsafe system and on whom no blame should be directed. James Reason, who first articulated the algorithm (described previously), is clear when describing his model that blaming individuals for events beyond their control, although it might be a salve to patient angst or satisfy the legal issues about accountability, does not fix a problem or make a system safer. This is a model of accountability which says we can look patients, regulators, purchasers, and each other in the face and say, "the people delivering care here are capable, conscientious and working hard to do the right thing."[28] This model allows quickly separating individual issues from system ones. What is critical is creating a safe environment that allows good nurses, doctors, and others to tell us when they make mistakes or have near misses.

Tragic examples highlight the need for this objective and clear evaluation mechanism as evidenced by the overdoses in Indianapolis in 2006 of the blood thinner, heparin. After the wrong concentration of heparin, 100 times too concentrated, was put in the automated pharmacy dispensing machine, nine very skilled individuals—six newborn intensive care unit nurses and three neonatologists—mistakenly took the wrong concentration of drug and administered it to very small infants. Three fatalities resulted.[29]

A similar episode occurred in 2007 involving the actor, Dennis Quaid, and his family in Los Angeles.[30] The media coverage of the Quaid's cases has highlighted their trauma as patients and the outrage that occurs when patients feel they are not being told the truth. Missing, as often is the case in general media stories, are the processes required to identify the underlying causes and fixes of these errors. They require an engineering and systematic approach that begins with an objective view of the events and from which flow insights about systematic flaws and individual culpability.

Thought leaders on both sides of the Atlantic have developed schema to address this topic. James Reason, in the early 1990s, described his incident analysis tree.[27] In the past decade David Marx developed his Just Culture Algorithm for evaluating the choices made by frontline providers, which incorporates and expands on Reason's work.[31] In both cases, the goal is to ensure appropriate accountability and an environment where every decision made by senior leadership and middle management passes a "sniff test" of integrity and ethics.

Regarding levels of culpability in some serious patient injuries, there are contributing factors for which agreement is universal. There are other individual actions or events that require careful analysis, teasing away bias or misconception, to arrive at a conclusion that the majority find fair and just. These are the gray areas in the analysis, lacking the discrete black and white forms and shapes that, if always present, would make this process much more straightforward.

The advantage of promoting, nurturing, and supporting a climate perceived as fair is that it opens the doors for discussion about problems and makes it acceptable to explore opportunities for improvement and to disagree and find resolution through testing and the quest for continuous improvement. In truth, a culture of fairness is a fundamental to the implementation of a safe system. And although not necessarily foremost on an operating room nurse's mind as he or she brings a patient into an operating room, a fair and just culture is omnipresent every time this occurs, and in part determines the degree to which the environment supports the safety of each procedure.

AN ENVIRONMENT OF ENTHUSIASM FOR TEAMWORK

Debriefing is a teamwork behavior that marries team practice and improvement.

There are only a few core team behaviors. An unlikely one to start with, but ultimately one of the most important, is debriefing. This one practice alone, if conducted routinely in a unit with the appropriate structural supports as described so far, would make surgical procedures safer.

Debriefing is the simple practice of convening a team immediately after finishing a procedure (or a series of procedures) to ask and answer three simple questions:

- What did we do well?
- What could we have done better?
- Did we learn anything that we should take into account for the next procedure?

If performed well, the debriefing, with experience and an agreed-on protocol, can generate essential information in under 120 seconds, all of 2 minutes. Once a debriefing discussion has occurred, the next set of steps, those that support the debriefing act, ultimately are more important than the debriefing itself; this is the phase in which the information is funneled to the unit so that an improvement process can be considered and its findings acted on.

Debriefings and the supporting structure are simple concepts but often are hard to put into practice. They require engaged and knowledgeable leadership, team buy-in, and the ability to analyze information and formulate process improvement actions. Debriefings and the supporting structure make the difference between a stellar unit and a mediocre one. The process is so important that every unit or clinical department should articulate a core value to describe it and then establish norms of conduct shaped by that value. The value could be stated as simply as endless learning and the norm of conduct an expectation that every team member is expected to participate in the debriefing. The expectations of leadership shine brightest here. If team members do not take on the expected norms of conduct, a series of proscribed steps must be followed that ultimately, and only if necessary, lead to the removal of that team member. This is not for the faint of heart to undertake. For leaders who want to be effective, it is essential.

Worthy of mention is Amy Edmondson's observations of operating room teams implementing what at the time was an innovative and new procedure—minimally invasive cardiac surgery.[32,33] The groups most effective were those for whom debriefing was a natural component of the ongoing minute-by-minute team function. This perspective is helpful in that it highlights the need for an environment that promotes continuous learning. It also serves to highlight another facet of learning, which is the infrastructure that captures concerns and insights and takes action to ameliorate problems and concerns.

Determining how to make debriefings a natural part of clinical environments is not part of most clinicians' thinking. Most clinical environments are not configured to undertake debriefings primarily because there is insufficient appreciation of their value, a paucity of understanding about how to do them efficiently, and incomplete knowledge of what to do with the information. Productivity-centered units and departments leave little to no time for even the briefest reflection. In fact, if time is taken to debrief, it usually is in the aftermath of a severe adverse event, and even then, it is conducted in a manner not likely to generate the best results.

Evaluations of severe adverse events should be conducted as closely as possible to the time of the event. After 24 hours, the minds of participants begin to fill in memory's blank or gray areas, reshaping the events to meet all manner of personal predispositions, to help protect oneself or explain away the uncomfortable.[34] Effective debriefing occurs at the most critical times only if it is practiced in the most mundane of times—in the debriefings that occur after a day's normal and successful activities. Daily, routine debriefings provide the opportunity to highlight the good work done by a team and group and always create the opportunity to learn something about how to make the work better.

Operating rooms in the United Kingdom, United States, and Canada are experimenting with debriefing as part of team training efforts and through collaboratives run by the IHI.[13] Almost every site is struggling with aspects of the debriefing, beginning with the question of when to do them. Most of those who have been successful have settled, to begin with, on a debriefing process that occurs in general anesthetics between the start of skin closure and patient emergence. There is no ideal time for this activity to occur, and this is true of that period; however, during this time, all the operating room participants tend to be together and usually there is a moment of stability and calm before the patient emerges. Remember that the debriefing discussion, if done well, can be as brief as 120 seconds. If well coordinated and if each member of the team understands its purpose, the debriefing can yield an extraordinary amount of information.

For a moment, consider a culture in which debriefing is fully developed and routinely practiced. In such cases, members of the team might, in real time, notice aspects of the procedure that are worthy of mention and tuck them away until the debriefing takes place. The result is a rapid debriefing discussion about things that went exceptionally well and should be repeated, those that were problematic and need to be fixed, and insights that might be fodder for future improvement tests. In such a setting, because the team members are used to the debriefing drill, they know who gets to speak up first (usually the most junior member or the individual who has the least authority), and they know how to express the issues and in what order. There also is a person assigned the responsibility of collecting the information on a form, which in a well-developed scenario is readily and easily accessible, and that individual—surgeon, nurse, technician, or anesthesia practitioner—knows where to deposit the form. Team members also know that the form serves a useful purpose, that the comments noted on the form are evaluated by departmental leaders, and that the comments are taken seriously. They know this because they see changes take place as a result of the comments and because they receive direct feedback when a specific comment they have made is acted on. For that feedback to occur, the well-designed collection instrument has a place for individual names so that leaders know where the comments originate, which procedures are being commented on, and what time of day the comments are made. This does not mean that every form must have all of this information; if a provider decides to pick up a form and insert an anonymous comment, that is acceptable, too. The culture is one of fairness so that providers are not hesitant about adding their names to the concerns expressed by others.

THE GOOD HEALTH CARE TEAM

What is a good health care team? A good team is a group of interdependent individuals who have the following characteristics.[35,36]

- They have diverse skills and share a common goal.
- Their output through synergy is greater than the sum of the individuals within the group.
- They have an appreciation of the roles played by each team member, including the leaders.
- They know each other's expertise so well that team members know where to turn to solve a problem.
- They have each agreed, individually, on norms of conduct, one of which is non-negotiable mutual respect.
- They address technical problems directly using the skill mix of the team but face complex problems that require adaptation and flexibility through collaboration and open discussion.

- Individuals may express concerns without fear of retribution and know that their concerns will engender only two possible responses: their concerns will be acted on or knowledge will be respectfully brought to light that mitigates the concern.

Excellent teams have team leaders who clarify, each time the team comes together, the expected norms of conduct. In addition to having agreed-on norms of conduct, outstanding teams have the added support of organizational endorsement.

TEAM LEADERS: THE CRITICAL ROLE OF LEADERSHIP

The active and committed engagement of executive and clinical leaders in systematically improving safety and quality is essential. One of the greatest challenges is aligning the frequently large number of strategic priorities in an organization with a simple, focused message that resonates with front-line clinicians caring for patients. Alignment and clarity of an organization's patient safety goals and work is critical. Senior leaders need to clearly message the priority of safe and reliable care and model these behaviors on a daily basis. Effective leaders continually reinforce the values and "this is the way we provide care within our organization." Excellent examples of how to do this well come from the messaging at Ascension Health to everyone working in their 71 hospitals: "Healthcare that works. Healthcare that is safe. Healthcare that leaves no one behind."[37] or from the longstanding Mayo Clinic motto that goes back to Dr. Mayo himself, "The needs of the patient come first."[38]

In Ascension's case, every organizational priority and activity filters through and aligns with those three goals, and providers, through internal activities, internal marketing, and time to reflect, know them. There is real value in every employee knowing and working toward a short list of clear goals every day. That's what habitually excellent organizations do.

Leaders also are keepers and drivers of the organizational culture. Setting the tone of how the organization values its people and how it treats them and expects them to treat each other is at the core of organizational excellence, or the lack thereof. The presence of overt disrespect is extremely destructive within a culture. Unfortunately, this behavior is pervasive in most health care systems and creates unacceptable risk, as nurses may be hesitant to call certain physicians with patient concerns because of the way they have been treated in the past. Sadly, hesitancy

to voice a concern or approach certain individuals is a common factor in serious episodes of avoidable patient harm.[16] Encouragingly, there is now a growing list of leaders and hospitals that are dealing directly with this issue. If they do not, they pay with increased nursing turnover, poorer patient satisfaction, and increased clinical risk.

Team leadership is not an innate skill; it is learned.[39] Physicians, one and all, are by definition most frequently the leaders of their teams, and nowhere is this truer than in the environments where surgery is performed. Equally true, however, is that the best decisions about direction and goals, those decisions that are most likely to support reliability and safety, accrue from a shared leadership between surgeon, anesthesiologist, nursing, and other team members and are feasible only with forethought, discussion about agreed-on norms of behavior, and practice.

One act of good leadership is to take the team through a process called briefing. Unlike terms, such as "pause" or "time-out," briefing is not a static, one-time event. Briefing is an ongoing process that ensures that all team members have a similar mental model of the team's game plan and presumes that as the plan changes or requires changing, team members will be informed and engaged in making informed decisions.

Briefings in operating rooms are multistep affairs, ideally beginning with a coming together of the surgical team with the patient in the preoperative area and a discussion that engages the patient and team members in delineating a game plan for that procedure. The briefing process might continue after the patient is sedated or asleep in the operating room, at which point a further briefing might ensue about any issues that team members might consider unsettling. These might include, for example, concerns about equipment logistics or a team member's personal comments about what he or she believes are their limitations that day, stated as a request that other team members work more closely with him or her. In the United States, a third part of the briefing process occurs just before incision and is the time-out. This is a regulatory requirement to ensure correct laterality of the procedure and identification of the patient and procedure.[40]

A good initial briefing process has four components in which leaders

- Ensure that all team members know the game plan.
- Assure team members they are operating in an environment of psychologic safety[41,42] where they may be completely comfortable speaking up about their concerns.

- Remind team members of agreed-on norms of conduct,[36] such as specific forms of communication that increase the likelihood of accurate transmission and reception of information.
- Expect excellence and excellent performance.[43] Reminding team members of their responsibility to do their best and remain, throughout, engaged in the performance of the team activity and centered on the game plan and team goals.

A briefing is only as good as the team leader who runs the briefing and, in general, physicians are not trained to do them nor have they trained health care frontline providers to participate in them.

The result in operating rooms is likely to be self-evident to every practitioner reading this article: the classic experience of anesthesiologists and surgeons schooled to believe in individual autonomy and the presumption of excellence, which leads to the scenario of the anesthesia provider, nurse, and technician arriving in an empty room and setting up their equipment. Then, at the appointed time, or often delayed and later, a nurse and anesthesia provider enter with a patient, at which time a dance begins between the nurse, anesthesia practitioner, and patient to gather the appropriate data and position the patient for anesthesia. Sometime during this process, or soon after, the surgeon or specialist arrives and may or may not acknowledge the presence of other team members, his or her behavior scripted on the assumption that all in the room are expert in their fields and that if they do what they are supposed to do the job will get safely done. Discussion is limited and, if there is any, it often relates to issues unrelated to the procedure, once again because of the assumption that everyone knows his or her job so that discussion about the work is redundant, might be an affront to the skills of the practitioners, or a waste of time. Nothing could be further from the truth.

Briefings, even with team members who work together daily and regularly, are necessary to remind team members of the values, norms of conduct, and practical game plan of every case. There are no shortcuts. Achieving a commonly understood game plan requires a robust briefing process by engaged leaders and team members.

Most agree that the time when the briefing process is truly useful is during critical events, when a patient is most in danger of harm.[44] Extraordinary in this common insight is the lack of understanding that to do this well in critical situations, it must be routine, commonplace, and excellently performed during the many common and straightforward procedures done daily in operating locations.[45] This simple concept has face validity that transcends the common naysayer's request for data to prove it. There is an entire science, however, underlying individual and group expertise that acknowledges that improvement occurs with practice of specific aspects within a skill set.[46] This same logic applies specifically to the perioperative setting.

Operating rooms and especially surgical nursing departments can and should set standards for briefings and have as a requirement for nursing participation in these areas that every case begin with a briefing. This should apply in every surgical procedure—operating rooms or interventional sites, such as radiology or gastroenterology. Whether or not the leader of a briefing is an anesthesia provider, nurse, or surgeon is open for discussion, depending on the experience of the group in performing all the components of a good briefing. These decisions may be made practically, based on the size of the provider groups who bring their care and the effort entailed to train the groups. Who initiates the briefing is less important than that the disciplines agree on and establish the expected norms of conduct for each and every procedure performed in that location. The end result will be greater participation in team practice, greater likelihood that all know the game plan, and, when combined with effective debriefings, a robust environment for continuous learning.

COMMUNICATION

There are three simple communication techniques that increase the likelihood that transmission and reception of information occur accurately and in a timely fashion.[47,48]

Closing the Loop

Closing the loop, also known as readback or hearback, is the simple technique of repeating back verbally what is requested or described in a manner that assures accurate comprehension. In technical conversations, the process is simple. "I need furosemide 10 mg please" receives a response of "furosemide 10 mg." Note that the hearback in this case does not have to include a "thank you" or any other reflexive social response. The agreed-on norm of conduct is a succinct repeat back devoid of extraneous words. Closing the loop in this way requires other agreed-on norms. For example, requests by a surgeon to a surgical technician for a particular instrument may require no verbal response if the placement of the instrument in the appropriate place—such as the surgeon's hand—is obvious. It is likely, however, that unusual requests always should have a closing of the loop to ensure mutual understanding.

Closing the loop is equally important in complex descriptions, such as the history of a patient during a handoff or when a surgeon is describing a patient and procedure to an anesthesiologist, anesthesia provider, nurse, or technician. Closing the loop entails a brief readback of the information imparted to ensure the receiving practitioner understands what has been described.

SBAR

A second communication form that promotes critical thinking and frames actions to be taken is a structured communication called SBAR (Situation, Background, Assessment, Recommendation). In departments where SBAR is used extensively, individuals can frame the conversation by actually saying, "I'm going to give you an SBAR," thereby telegraphing to the recipient the order of the information about to be imparted. The Situation is equivalent to the headline in a newspaper. It should be designed to be brief, succinct, and capture the attention of the recipient. In a crisis situation, "The situation is that we've lost 300 mL of blood in the last few minutes" is an example of a clear and concerning situation statement.

Background follows in which a slightly more expansive background is given to explain the situation. "The blood loss increased when the abdomen was cranked open, the retractor tucked further under the liver, and you started to suction further down in the abdomen."

Assessment is the evaluation or critical thinking par, and is one of SBAR's strengths in that it promotes the analysis of contributing and causative factors that may help all team members focus on the problem at hand. "I know you've been mopping up in the abdomen but this bleeding seems excessive. I don't know the problem but I'm concerned." In and of itself the concern is enough to warrant the discussion and is a reasonable assessment if a team member's gut feeling is the only precipitant for the SBAR.

The Recommendation further drives critical thinking: "Are you looking for a bleeding site and should I call for blood to the OR?" The surgeon may know or see something that the nurse or anesthesia provider does not and at this point add or alter the suggested actions. Regardless, the SBAR format clarifies for all a structured process of thinking and information sharing. When done well it also promotes learning.

Critical Language

The third communication technique is critical language, an agreed-on phrase that stops activity, described in other industries as "stopping the line." When a team member perceives a risk and believes that there is limited time to address it, a critical phrase is a useful and powerful mechanism to gain attention of all team members and momentarily stop all activity. Agreeing on a term may help a junior team member overcome the hesitancy to speak up or the common problem of speaking up indirectly and possibly delaying needed quick action. Many obstetric units now use the term, "I need clarity," as the critical statement known to all team members; its use stops activity so that a group evaluation may be made of the perceived risk. In the obstetrics setting, when every patient is alert and aware and families are often in attendance, the term also is neutral so as to not cause unnecessary alarm.

The test of effective teams and leaders occurs not only when a concern is real, because then action is obvious and the team member who picked up the problem is congratulated, but also when a concern is inaccurate—that is when the real test of teamwork and leadership occurs. The response by other team members in the latter case really determines the health of the team and whether or not the environment in the future will be a learning, supportive, and reliable one. Intolerance of team members when they speak up and are wrong is a sure mechanism to decrease the likelihood they will speak up in the future.

This should not be misconstrued as a requirement to tolerate mediocrity. If individuals repeatedly misunderstand or misrepresent a situation, then it is entirely possible that they need remediation or are in the wrong position. Well-functioning teams are cognizant of the difference between excellent evaluation of concerns that sometimes are wrong and incompetent evaluations that slow the team from doing its work. As long as the actions taken are appropriate, discussed openly, and pass a general "sniff test" of reasonableness by team members, the environment for outstanding team practice will remain viable.

SITUATION AWARENESS AND CONFLICT RESOLUTION

Conflict is an intrinsic part of teamwork.[34] A team's synergy derives from the inputs of each team member and the ineffable combining of perspectives and efforts to produce a sum greater than the individual parts. The strength of a team comes from the ability to evaluate, reconcile, combine, and mesh these perspectives into a viewpoint that uses the best of all. Along the way, it is likely that team members occasionally will feel strongly—and differently—and find themselves in conflict about the team's game plan. Much of the time these differences are grist for great relationships, and team members likely will appreciate the reconciliation process as it often is educational. Occasionally differences of opinion flare into disagreement, and the glue of the team membership is tested. At these times, hierarchy or strength of personality may determine the course of action rather than what is in the best interest of the patient. Formalized practices to manage conflict can help ensure that the best course of action prevails. An adage that is helpful is, "the sun never sets on a disagreement between two team members." In other words, departments should have a codified mechanism for conflict resolution, committed to by all team members, to sit down with those they argue with to resolve the issues as a regular and required course of daily action. This is a true test of leadership because many of the serious discussions in this setting are unlikely to be successful if left solely to the two team members who disagree. A moderator often is necessary, a leader who has the formal authority and the informal respect to facilitate a discussion that leads to resolution or clearing the air.

Norms of conduct about challenging team members can help in this regard, and rules of engagement can be agreed on as a departmental or organizational expectation. Members of the department must agree to abide by these constructs, and department leaders must be willing to censure those who do not follow them. An important part of making these conduct norms real is gaining open commitment by all department members that they will abide by them. This may entail public commitment in departmental meetings and the signing of a document where the norms of conduct are described.

One challenge rule that has shown promise as a mechanism to resolve disagreements is a set of escalating challenges which, if they do not resolve the differences, lead to collaboration with others. One set is to use the words, curious, concerned, challenge, collaborate. If a team member is troubled by a course of action taken by another team member, he or she might say, "I'm curious why you've chosen this particular course of action." In departments where the challenge rules are understood, the recipient might realize that the team member addressing them has started a challenge process. If the response does not satisfy the team member's curiosity, he or she might next say, "I'm concerned about the course of action

we're taking." This ups the ante in the challenge, and the recipient should now clearly appreciate that a negotiation needs to occur if a further challenge is to be avoided. If the response does not alleviate the concern, the team member may move up to the third level of challenge and say, "I'm not comfortable with this course of action and I feel I have to challenge it." If circumstances permit, this challenge should lead to a set of prescribed actions, the primary one being involving a third party who has the expertise or objectivity to help resolve the difference of opinion. It may be necessary to identify who these arbiters are, although in some groups it may be adequate that any other member of the team be called on to help.

The department would have to agree on a mechanism to help the two team members resolve their differences should an arbiter be unavailable. In some, hopefully infrequent, situations, a decision needs to be made rapidly or no third person is available, for example during middle-of-the-night emergency procedures. In that case, hierarchy or accountability for the patient may have to be the deciding factor, although departments might experiment with other, better solutions (a senior person is assigned responsibility for clinical and challenge situations, with the clear understanding that the threshold for calling is to be set at a very low level).

No solution takes into account every situation, but a formal and clear set of conduct norms pertaining to conflict resolution is essential to ensure that the inevitable deviation of behavior from norms that is intrinsic in each of us as a characteristic of humanness is managed effectively.

LEADERS ENGAGED IN SAFETY AND RELIABILITY THROUGH THE USE OF DATA

The components of reliability and team practice that support safe care require leadership engagement before implementation; all leaders must understand the concepts well enough to explain them to others—concepts they believe are important enough to make them foundational to further action.

Presuming that there is agreement to move forward, education and practice are necessary if safety is to flourish; without ongoing effort, including practice, measurement, and continuous learning, the practices described in this article are likely to extinguish—even in those departments that perceive them to be of intrinsic value. They consume some time and require a continuously different paradigm than is current in health care today and a kind of reflection that many individuals avoid for many complex reasons. Team excellence requires organizational and individual concentration.

A powerful measure that, if used wisely, leaders will find essential is the measurement of safety culture within an operating room, hospital, or health care system. Evaluation of provider attitudes toward safety, teamwork, management, and improvement offer a valuable perspective on the strengths and weaknesses of specific clinical care areas and the relationships between care providers. Further, if they can not be measured, how can they be managed? The Safety Attitudes Questionnaire[49] is one widely used and validated instrument that has been used in more than 2000 hospitals. Hospitals can measure safety culture at a clinical unit level and then map these units and compare them with specific high-risk clinical areas: obstetrics, surgery, critical care, emergency medicine, oncology, and areas identified by claims and injury within the hospital from their own data. Interventions in each clinical unit then can be chosen to strengthen specific weaknesses and safety culture tracked over time, in combination with other operational or outcome measures, to follow improvement. Between safety culture and direct observation, another measurement tool becoming increasingly well understood, organizations now have powerful tools to engage clinical teams in constructive dialog about their strengths in and barriers to delivering optimal care. Feeding back this information is a powerful driver to help improve team cultures over time. The development of Web-based platforms to allow easy safety culture data entry, analysis, and report generation is an active area of interest and research. In the coming years, health care and health care culture, like every other sector, will become ever more illuminated by metrics.

HEALTH LITERACY

Health literacy is the ability of patients and their families to understand the process and goals of their medical care. Awareness and consistent approaches to this issue can have a huge impact on the quality and safety of clinical care. Large numbers of patients are at risk. There are five levels of health literacy. Virtually all the readers of this article are level 5—quite literate. Approximately 20% of the American population is level 1, which means they have a difficult time reading the headlines of a newspaper. Many others are level 2, which means they have difficulty reading a bar graph, interpreting a bus schedule, or understanding a pie chart on the front page of *USA Today*. In major metropolitan United States markets, 40% to 70% of the population is literacy level

2 or below. They are seriously at risk for having lower health status and increased costs.

There are some simple tools that are effective and available through the American Medical Association.[50] The first technique is Ask Me 3,[51] which means that every patient and their family members should leave a medical encounter with knowledge of three key aspects of their care: What is my basic medical or surgical problem? Why is it important I know this? and What needs to happen for me to get better? The second technique is called a teach-back. Instead of asking, "Do you know what we talked about?" and having them politely nod their heads if they understand or not (and often they do not), we now ask, "You've heard us talk about this; please take a moment and tell me how you'll explain this to your family." This closed-loop technique greatly increases the chances that patients and their families actually do understand the process and goals of their medical care. This is impressively low-hanging fruit in the quest to improving medical care. Gail Nielsen and her colleagues at Iowa Health System have done probably the most comprehensive implementation program on health literacy.[52] They have systematic training for all their clinical staff, during which patients who have had literacy issues share their stories with clinical staff.

DISCLOSING UNANTICIPATED ADVERSE EVENTS/JUST CULTURE

An ethical environment and one that is considered just and fair also must include the ability to have honest, open conversations with patients and their families in the aftermath of an adverse event. Most doctors, nurses, and hospital leaders traditionally have had little or no formal training in having these difficult conversations at times that are major life experiences for vulnerable patients in the aftermath of harm. There is an increasing body of evidence that having the capability of skilled individuals to facilitate open, honest discussions in the aftermath of an adverse event not only provides much better care but also greatly reduces the risk for lawsuits.[53–55]

COPIC, the largest malpractice carrier in Colorado, has had an early intervention program for the past several years through which physicians are incentivized by premium reductions to report within 24 hours any adverse event or negative patient interaction. COPIC then uses skilled personnel to reach out directly to patients and their families to see how they can help support and, when feasible, resolve the situation. These personnel are trained to be supportive, to ensure that the patients believe they have a straightforward ally to work with and that they will not be abandoned by their health care provider as a result of the disagreement or mishap. If patients want an attorney, they have to drop out of the program. They have resolved more than 3000 cases, writing a check to one in four patients for an average of approximately $5000. Only seven patients have dropped out and retained lawyers; two have filed suits.[56]

Kaiser Permanente has a national ombudsman mediator program adopted from the National Naval Medical Center in Bethesda, Maryland. There are trained ombudsman mediators in almost all Kaiser hospitals whose job is to take care of clinicians, patients, and their family members in the aftermath of an adverse outcome. These individuals report directly to the CEO in each hospital, and centrally to Kaiser Risk Management, to ensure clarity of reporting and minimize the likelihood that their actions will be influenced by the priorities of hospital departments. Their goal is to be an impartial advocate so that parties involved can engage in a productive dialog that helps resolve the issues. This program has been well received by all parties, and early indications are that it probably helps reduce claims.

SUMMARY

For many reasons, health care overall has been slow to adopt the reliability engineering well known for decades to other industries. National health care systems have their own reasons and in each and every one there are confounding factors that blind leadership and physicians to many of the threads listed. In the United States, the primary problem is in the methods of reimbursement because payment has been unrelated to quality or safety.[57]

Although prescient and leading-edge health systems are moving forward, there are many pockets of resistance and significant parts of the United States health system have not started down this path, but the general trend is likely to favor those who adapt to the new paradigm—because outcomes are now measurable, benchmarking increasingly is associated with pay for performance, and increasingly well-coordinated consumerism favors well-organized and forward thinking groups.

In summary, comprehensive patient safety and quality solutions share fundamental principles. They tend to require a holistic framework that is part of a core strategy, a carefully constructed structural framework that matches the strategic goals, and where execution occurs at a variety of levels.

First, changing the culture of patient safety through leadership engagement and team training ensures that people across hospitals and health care systems are more likely to achieve the goals required for safe and reliable care. The success of technology implementation is equally dependent on effective leadership engagement and teamwork, and, if well implemented, these efforts go further than improving safety and technology; they mitigate clinical, operational, and financial risk by improving organizational ability to makes all types of needed changes.

Second, healthy patient safety solutions should be measurable, unit specific, dynamic, and risk adjusted. Cultural assessment, measures obtained through direct observation, and actions tracked as a component of learning to action cycles all aid in assessing patient safety milieu.

Third, all our work is for patients and should be patient focused. Patients must be considered team members and, to ensure comprehension of their clinical problems, health literacy concepts applied. At the same time, they are our patients—which requires effective disclosure policies be used to support them and clinicians when care goes wrong.

Fourth, the ideal approach in managing cost-effective safety programs is to deliver the best in clinical practice and scientific rigor in a manner that scales across large organizations and networks. The only way to ensure ongoing improvement is knowing how to spread change in a standardized manner where providers, through cycles of learning, can speak up about their insights and concerns and see actions generated as a result. A just culture increases the likelihood that individuals will speak up.

And, fifth, because changing culture demands judgment and takes time, programs that draw on leading clinical expertise and sustainable operational modeling are likely to deliver safe and reliable care—especially when flourishing under the disciplines of ongoing assessment, action, and accountability.

Increasingly, precise invasive treatments performed as part of prescriptive protocols achieve, when performed well, targeted and reliable results. This trend ensures increasing operating room complexity. A culture of reliability is not optional, it is essential, and today we have the knowledge to achieve it.

REFERENCES

1. Ginsburg PB, Pham HH, McKenzie K, et al. Distorted payment system undermines business case for

health quality and efficiency gains. Issue Brief Cent Stud Health Syst Change 2007;112:1–4.

2. Baker DP, Salas E, King H, et al. The role of teamwork in the professional education of physicians: current status and assessment recommendations. Jt Comm J Qual Patient Saf 2005;31: 185–202.

3. Mallon B. Ernest amory codman: the end result of a life in medicine. 1st edition. New York (NY): W.B. Saunders Company; 2000.

4. Brennan TA, Leape LL, Laird NM, et al. Incidence of adverse events and negligence in hospitalized patients: results of the Harvard Medical Practice Study I. N Engl J Med 1991;324:370–6.

5. Leape LL, Brennan TA, Laird N, et al. The nature of adverse events in hospitalized patients: results of the Harvard Medical Practice Study II. N Engl J Med 1991;324:377–84.

6. Kohn LT, Corrigan J, Donaldson MS. To err is human: building a safer health system. Washington, DC: National Academy Press; 2000.

7. Delbanco SF, Suzanne F. Delbanco on the leapfrog group and employer purchasing power. interview by Pamela K. Scarrow. J Healthc Qual 2004;26:18–21.

8. Eliminating serious, preventable, and costly medical. errors-never events. Available at: http://www.cms. hhs.gov/apps/media/press/factsheet.asp?Counter= 1863&;;intNumPerPage=10&checkDate=&checkKey=& srchType=1&numDays=3500&srchOpt=0&srchData=& keywordType=All&chkNewsType=6&intPage=&showAll= &pYear=&year=&desc=false&cboOrder=date.Accessed July 23, 2008 2008.

9. Aetna won't pay for never events. Wall Str J 2008;. Available at: http://online.wsj.com/article/SB1200 35439914089727.html. Accessed January 15, 2008.

10. Beth Israel Deaconess Medical Center. Our awards & recognition: Beth Israel Deaconess Medical Center—Boston, hospital, quality, awards, recognition, best hospital, safety. Available at: http://www.bidmc. harvard.edu/display.asp?node_id=8345. 2008; Accessed July 23, 2008.

11. MDH Division of Health Policy. Adverse health events reporting law: minnesota's 28 reportable events—minnesota dept. of health. Available at: http://www.health. state.mn.us/patientsafety/ae/adverse27events.html. 2008. Accessed July 23, 2008.

12. Ableson R. In bid for better care, surgery with a warranty—New York Times. Available at: http:// www.nytimes.com/2007/05/17/business/17quality. html. Accessed July 23, 2008.

13. Institute for healthcare improvement: home. Available at: http://www.ihi.org/ihi. Accessed July 23, 2008.

14. Cooper JB, Gaba D. No myth: anesthesia is a model for addressing patient safety. Anesthesiology 2002; 97:1335–7.

15. Eichhorn JH, Cooper JB, Cullen DJ, et al. Anesthesia practice standards at Harvard: a review. J Clin Anesth 1988;1:55–65.

16. Leonard MS, Frankel A, Simmonds T, et al. Achieving safe and reliable healthcare: strategies and solutions (management series). 1st edition. Chicago: Health Administration Press; 2004.

17. Marx D. Patient safety and the "just culture": a primer for health care executives. New York: Columbia University: Trustees of Columbia University in the City of New York; 2001.

18. Marx D. How building a 'just culture' helps an organization learn from errors. OR Manager 2003;19(1): 14–5.

19. Frankel A, Graydon-Baker E, Neppl C, et al. Patient safety leadership walkrounds. Jt Comm J Qual Saf 2003;29:16–26.

20. Frankel A, Grillo SP, Baker EG, et al. Patient safety leadership walkrounds at partners healthcare: learning from implementation. Jt Comm J Qual Patient Saf 2005;31:423–37.

21. Yates GR, Hochman RF, Sayles SM, et al. Sentara Norfolk General Hospital: accelerating improvement by focusing on building a culture of safety. Jt Comm J Qual Saf 2004;30:534–42.

22. Spear SJ. Learning to lead at Toyota. Harv Bus Rev 2004;82:78–86, 151.

23. Liker JK, Hoseus M. Center for quality people and organizations . Toyota culture: the heart and soul of the toyota way. New York: McGraw-Hill; 2008.

24. Liker JK. The toyota way: 14 management principles from the world's greatest manufacturer. New York: McGraw-Hill 2004.

25. Mohr JJ, Batalden PB. Improving safety on the front lines: the role of clinical microsystems. Qual Saf Health Care 2002;11:45–50.

26. Freiberg K, Freiberg J. Nuts! Southwest airlines' crazy recipe for business and personal success. 1st trade pbk. edition. New York: Broadway Books; 1998.

27. Reason JT. Managing the risks of organizational accidents. Aldershot, Hampshire (England): Ashgate; 1997.

28. Reason JT. Managing the risks of organizational accidents. In: Aldershot, Hants, England. Brookfield (VT): Ashgate; 1997.

29. Family wants medicine label changed after preemie deaths—staying healthy news story—WRTV indianapolis. Available at: http://www.theindychannel. com/health/9903031/detail.html; 2008. Accessed July 23, 2008.

30. FOXNews.com—Dennis Quaid's twins among three newborns given drug overdose—celebrity gossip | entertainment news | arts and entertainment. Available at: http://www.foxnews.com/story/ 0,00.html. 2933, 312357. Accessed July 23, 2008.

31. Marx D. How building a "just culture" helps an organization learn from errors. OR Manager 2003;19:1, 14–5, 20.

32. Edmondson AC, Wooley AW. Understanding outcomes of organizational learning interventions. In: Easterby-Smith M, Lyles MA, editors. The blackwell handbook of organizational learning and knowledge management (Blackwell handbooks in management). Malden (MA): Wiley-Blackwell; 2003. p. 696.

33. Edmondson AC. Learning from failure in health care: frequent opportunities, pervasive barriers. Qual Saf Health Care 2004;13(Suppl 2):ii3–9.

34. Schacter DL. The seven sins of memory: how the mind forgets and remembers. Boston: Houghton Mifflin; 2001.

35. Salas E, Swezey RW. Teams: their training and performance. Norwood (NJ): Ablex Publ; 1992.

36. Hackman JR. Groups that work (and those that don't): creating conditions for effective teamwork. San Francisco (CA): Jossey-Bass; 1990.

37. Pryor DB, Tolchin SF, Hendrich A, et al. The clinical transformation of ascension health: eliminating all preventable injuries and deaths. Jt Comm J Qual Patient Saf 2006;32:299–308.

38. Davidson JH. The committed enterprise. Oxford: Butterworth-Heinemann; 2002.

39. Heifetz RA. Leadership without easy answers. Cambridge (MA): Belknap Press of Harvard University Press; 1994.

40. JCAHO. National patient safety goals and universal protocol for preventing wrong-site, wrong-procedure, and wrong-person surgery. Joint Commission for Accreditation of Hospitals Organization.

41. Roberto MA, Bohmer RM, Edmondson AC. Facing ambiguous threats. Harv Bus Rev 2006;84:106–13.

42. Bohmer RM, Edmondson AC. Organizational learning in health care. Health Forum J 2001;44:32–5.

43. Collins J. Good to great: why some companies make the leap—and others don't. London: Random House Business Books; 2001.

44. Marks MA, Zaccaro SJ, Mathieu JE. Performance implications of leader briefings and team-interaction training for team adaptation to novel environments. J Appl Psychol 2000;85:971–86.

45. Helmreich RL, Merritt AC, Wilhelm JA. The evolution of crew resource management training in commercial aviation. Int J Aviat Psychol 1999;9:19–32.

46. Ericsson KA. The Cambridge handbook of expertise and expert performance. New York: Cambridge University Press; 2006.

47. Gandhi TK, Graydon-Baker E, Huber CN, et al. Closing the loop: follow-up and feedback in a patient safety program. Jt Comm J Qual Patient Saf 2005; 31:614–21.

48. Leonard M, Graham S, Bonacum D. The human factor: the critical importance of effective teamwork and communication in providing safe care. Qual Saf Health Care 2004;13(Suppl 1):i85–90.

49. Sexton JB, Helmreich RL, Neilands TB, et al. The safety attitudes questionnaire: psychometric properties, benchmarking data, and emerging research. BMC Health Serv Res 2006;61–11.

50. NIFL-HEALTH 2002: [NIFL-HEALTH:3700] re: AMA'a health literacy. Available at: http://www.nifl.gov/nifl-health/2002/0197.html. 2008. Accessed July 23, 2008.

51. Mika VS, Wood PR, Weiss BD, et al. Ask me 3: improving communication in a hispanic pediatric outpatient practice. Am J Health Behav 2007; 31(Suppl 1):S115–21.

52. Ask me 3. Available at: http://www.npsf.org/askme3/PCHC. Accessed September 20, 2008.

53. Gallagher TH, Levinson W. Disclosing harmful medical errors to patients: a time for professional action. Arch Intern Med 2005;165:1819–24.

54. Gallagher TH, Studdert D, Levinson W. Disclosing harmful medical errors to patients. N Engl J Med 2007;356:2713–9.

55. Browning DM, Meyer EC, Truog RD, et al. Difficult conversations in health care: cultivating relational learning to address the hidden curriculum. Acad Med 2007;82:905–13.

56. Berlinger N. After harm: medical error and the ethics of forgiveness. Baltimore (MD): Johns Hopkins University Press; 2005.

57. Lee PR, LeRoy LB, Ginsberg PB, et al. Physician payment reform: an idea whose time has come. Med Care Rev 1990;47:137–63.

Using Human Factors to "Balance" Your Operating Room

Chasity Burrows Walters, MSN, RN[a], Aileen Killen, PhD, RN[a],*,
Jill Garrett, RN, CPHQ[b]

KEYWORDS

- Human factors • Ergonomics • Balance theory
- Patient safety

Health care is an inherently risky business, and with that risk errors are inevitable. Medical errors represent a public health issue that has been increasingly well recognized since the sentinel Institute of Medicine report[1] was published a decade ago. Since then, the demands on health care to redesign processes to ensure a safer system have been increasing. Despite the efforts of health care leaders, policy makers, and public health advocates, however, the number of errors continues to rise.[2] As one of the most complex work environments in health care,[3] the operating room (OR) is a common site for adverse events.[4] It involves teams of highly trained professionals interacting with advanced technology in high-risk situations, and the nature of such work places these industries at risk for errors.[4] The largest numbers of errors result from treatment provided in the OR.[5,6] The causes of these errors are variable and include technical errors[6,7] and communication deficiencies.[3,8,9]

Although surgical safety has long been a phenomenon of concern,[10] why do these errors persist? Safety in the operating room historically has been viewed as a matter of individual human factors. Although health care continued to perpetuate a culture of blame and shame, other industries successfully adopted a systems approach to errors. This approach has left the health care industry lagging behind other high-reliability industries, such as aviation, when it comes to designing safer systems. Shifting focus from the notion of errors resulting from human failure to errors as a consequence of the underlying systemic inefficiencies requires a change in thinking, and it is gaining momentum. This change is imperative to create and sustain health care environments conducive to patient safety. It requires, however, an understanding of work systems not traditionally taught to the nurses, surgeons, or allied health providers who are so well intentioned toward the pursuit of safety. This article provides an introduction to concepts used in a systems approach followed by strategies that can be implemented to cultivate a safer OR.

THE OPERATING ROOM AS A MICROSYSTEM

A work system is essentially any environment in which work is performed. In the OR, for example, the work system can be described as a microsystem in which small, interdependent groups of people work as a team to provide patient care. There the microsystem typically consists of 5 to 15 people, including the surgeon, assistants, anesthesia providers, scrub person, circulating nurse, unlicensed assistive personnel (eg, nursing assistants, equipment technicians, housekeeping personnel), perfusionists, monitoring technicians, and possibly others. The large number of participants gets further complicated by hierarchical issues within the system and the multiple handoffs that take place during a typical case. Although each member of the microsystem has a specific role, one

[a] Memorial Sloan Kettering Cancer Center, 160 East 53 Street, New York, NY 10022, USA
[b] Memorial Health System, 1400 E. Boulder Street, Colorado Springs, CO 80909, USA
* Corresponding author.
E-mail address: killena@mskcc.org (A. Killen).

Perioperative Nursing Clinics 3 (2008) 277–285
doi:10.1016/j.cpen.2008.08.009

member cannot function effectively without the support of others. Finally, this group needs to perform in routine situations and highly specialized or crisis situations. These factors describe some issues that occur daily in the OR that are not generally considered in their entirety in attempts to create a safe environment.

Viewing the OR as a microsystem provides a basis for understanding the complexity of systems, and this shifting of approach may allow for a significant decrease in errors.[11] From the systems perspective, errors are viewed as a consequence of a system breakdown rather than being caused by an individual working in the system. This thinking is fundamental to the field of human factors, which has been used in other complex industries to balance the components of work.[12]

HUMAN FACTORS

"Human factors" is an umbrella term that refers to the interaction of humans on and by the system in which humans work. Historically, the term "human factors" has been used in the United States, and the term "ergonomics" has been used in Europe. Much of the current literature uses the terms interchangeably. In fact, the Human Factors and Ergonomics Society uses the terms synonymously in their definition: "Ergonomics (or human factors) is the scientific discipline concerned with the understanding of interactions among humans and other elements of a system, and the profession that applies theory, principles, data, and other methods to design to optimize human well-being and overall system performance."[13] "Human factors" offers a way to understand the interactions among the elements of the work system, as opposed to addressing the elements individually. It takes into account human strengths and limitations with the goal of offering solutions that limit the dependence of the work system on less reliable human characteristics (ie, memory) and places greater emphasis on systems processes (ie, standardization).

In their study of work systems, Smith and Sainfort[14] developed the Balance Theory to conceptualize the interaction of five human factors components within the system: the individual, tasks, tools and technologies, environment, and organizational factors (**Fig. 1**). These components work together to create a "stress load" that challenges an individual's biological, psychologic, and behavioral resources.[15] These five components should be considered equally when designing a product, process, or system to achieve effective, efficient, and safe results. This article presents those human factor components as they relate to the OR and discusses how balancing all five factors within a work system can improve patient safety.

INDIVIDUAL

The characteristics of an individual in the work system include everything the perioperative nurse "brings" to work, including individual characteristics such as past experience, abilities, physical and emotional health, motivation, and professional aspirations. Many of these characteristics are not static. Fatigue, for example, has been implicated in errors in disasters such as Exxon Valdez oil spill, Chernobyl nuclear disaster, and Three Mile Island situation.[16] Adverse surgical outcomes have been linked to fatigue,[17] and although little is known specifically about the impact of fatigue on the practice of OR nursing, it presents some unique challenges.

In addition to working a full-time schedule, perioperative nurses often need to take call. Balancing work and personal obligations becomes more difficult, which can force nurses to work without adequate sleep. Lack of sleep impairs one's ability to deliver safe care. Research has shown that after 17 hours without sleep, performance is equivalent to having a blood alcohol level of 0.05%;[18] it further degrades to 0.10% after 24 hours without sleep.[19] Recognizing fatigue as an important factor in the OR, the Association of Perioperative Registered Nurses has issued a position statement based on an extensive review of the literature outlining recommendations for safe on-call practices.

Another individual characteristic that demands consideration in the designing of a safe OR is the experience level. Like other specialty nurses, perioperative nurses bring varying degrees of knowledge, skills, and experience to the OR. The gap between available experienced perioperative nurses and the needs of operating rooms around the country has required creative hiring and training practices by perioperative leaders. New graduate nurses and experienced nurses from other specialties are choosing perioperative nursing for their career paths. Compounded by the aging surgical patient population and the complexity of modern surgical interventions, orientation and ongoing skill development are crucial to balance the work environment. Addressing this issue, the Association of Perioperative Registered Nurses published a position statement on "Orientation of the Registered Professional Nurse to the Perioperative Setting," which provides suggested timelines for orientation of novice and experienced perioperative nurses. These guidelines provide justification

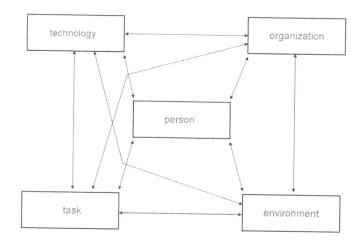

Fig. 1. Smith and Sainfort work system model. (*Adapted from* Smith MJ, Sainfort PC. A balance theory of job design for stress reduction. Int J Ind Econ 1989;4:75; with permission.)

for perioperative leaders as they request resources of time, staff, and money. The fallout of this phenomenon is complex; the need for ongoing preceptorship programs can burden the experienced staff who are adding this additional responsibility to their full workload. Training and development only go so far to facilitate transition to perioperative nursing. Novice perioperative nurses who have expertise in other clinical areas of practice also may require special support as they move from being "expert" nurses in one specialty to "novice" perioperative nurses.

Although this section focuses on particular individual human factors, including fatigue and experience, several other characteristics can be managed by targeting elements within the work system. Human factor limitations and error reduction strategies can be implemented to compensate for them:

- Humans have a limited short-term memory capacity, so use checklists to reduce reliance on memory.
- Sensory overload in the operating room requires staff to be constantly alert to everything around them. Limiting the availability of choices, such as by using unit dose medication whenever possible, can decrease the likelihood of a medication error.
- Cognitive tunnel vision can occur related to stress in high intense situations. Using forcing functions whenever possible, such as automatic shut-off valves on warming devices, can mitigate this risk.

TASK

According to the Balance Theory, the tasks of the work system affect and are impacted by the individual, technology, and the environment.[15] The tasks required in the OR must be considered to achieve a balanced work system, necessitating attention to concepts such as the appropriate use of skills, workload, and work pressures.

The ability to identify and prioritize the enormous number of individual tasks required of a perioperative nurse is a skill that evolves along the novice to expert continuum. Time pressures, combined with high-level multitasking, are routine. Nurses face significant competition for attention during routine and critical points in a surgical procedure.[3] The workload in the OR varies and is impacted by the need to retrieve additional resources, such as supplies and equipment, and the need to perform safety-related activities, such as "count" and handoff. The requirements of these tasks are physical and cognitive. Standardization and simplification should be the mantra for developing error reduction strategies for the task component of a balanced work system. As part of the "Safe Surgery Saves Lives" campaign, the World Health Organization (WHO) developed the WHO Surgical Safety Checklist, which can be used to remind the surgical team of key tasks to be performed in the preoperative, intraoperative, and immediate postoperative phases of care.[20]

Situational awareness, a concept borrowed from high reliability organizations,[21] allows members of the team to have an accurate understanding of "what's going on" and "what is likely to happen next." It allows the entire team to be on the same page. Institutions across the country are identifying ways to increase situational awareness in their operating rooms. Memorial Hospital in Colorado Springs, CO, identified briefings as the first step in creating situational awareness. The elements of briefing were determined by the Unit Practice Council and were designed into the current "count board," which offers the appropriate visual cue when in the OR scrubbed and standing at the table (**Fig. 2**). Electronic documentation of

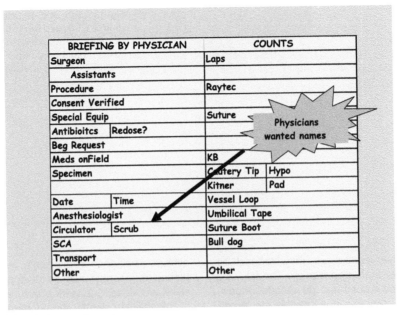

BRIEFING BY PHYSICIAN		COUNTS	
Surgeon		Laps	
Assistants			
Procedure		Raytec	
Consent Verified			
Special Equip		Suture	
Antibioitcs	Redose?		
Beg Request			
Meds onField		KB	
Specimen		Cautery Tip	Hypo
		Kitner	Pad
Date	Time	Vessel Loop	
Anesthesiologist		Umbilical Tape	
Circulator	Scrub	Suture Boot	
SCA		Bull dog	
Transport			
Other		Other	

Physicians wanted names

Fig. 2. Memorial hospital count board.

a physician-led briefing was later added to facilitate the collection of metrics for this process improvement (**Fig. 3**). Likewise, during the design and construction of their operating room platform, Memorial Sloan Kettering Cancer Center in New York launched the concept of the "Wall of Knowledge" (**Fig. 4**). One component of the "Wall of Knowledge" is the "OR Dashboard," which displays continuous real-time data to all members of the surgical team regarding patient information, the progress of the case, and team members.

In addition to these strategies involving task management and awareness, other error reduction strategies can be implemented to simplify tasks and processes:

- Support the most appropriate use of skills by considering the redistribution of work to ancillary personnel.
- Use checklists and automated reminders when possible to remind staff of critical activities. Multitasking can lead to errors.
- Decrease number of choices by using pre-packed custom procedure packs.
- Decrease number of steps necessary to complete a task. Design a pass-thru cabinet to obtain supplies from central core to operating room (which has the added value of decreasing the number of staff coming in and out of room).
- Reduce reliance on memory and experience by using up-to-date preference cards.

TECHNOLOGY

The modern operating room is a technologically sophisticated work environment. Battles and Keyes[22] described the relationship between technology and patient safety as a "two-edged sword." Technology can assist perioperative nurses by automating repetitive, time-consuming, and error-prone tasks, yet it may provide distractions and competition for attention. The addition of new technology can burden individuals who need to acquire new skills or who may be concerned about changes to their job functions as a result of adoption of new technology. The "two-edged sword" of new technologies[22] can be told in a "tale of two communication devices." When designing a new OR communication system at Memorial Sloan Kettering Cancer Center, a hands-free phone was selected for the nurses' documentation station. The phone plugged into a USB port on the computer. A surgeon picked up the phone at the end of the case to call a patient's family, and the phone number was entered in the nurses' documentation fields because the computer could not tell the difference between the phone and the keyboard. On the other hand, a hands-free wireless communication system[23] was implemented and was hugely successful in facilitating communication between anesthesia and nursing staff and nursing staff and support personnel.

Seeking technologic solutions is often thought to provide a simple answer to complex problems.

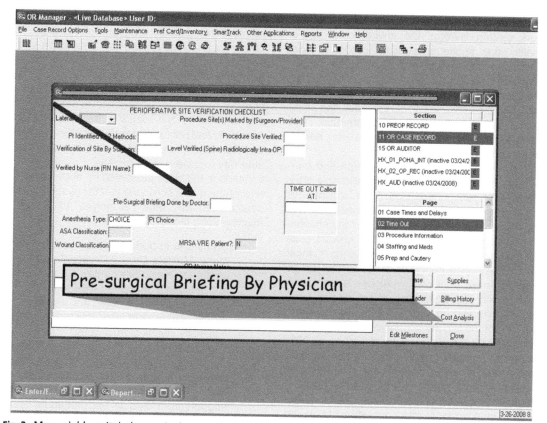

Fig. 3. Memorial hospital electronic documentation.

A wise colleague once said, "Never automate a broken system." Perioperative managers need to be mindful of the use of technology to "balance" the work system. Kukla and colleagues[24] suggested that safety concerns for automated systems should be a design that is easy to use and provides a better way for staff to do their work (or at least as good as current methods). Before implementation of any automated system, a detailed analysis of the current work flow should be undertaken. The Institute for Healthcare Improvement is an excellent resource when getting started with the documentation of a workflow.[25]

In this technological era, new tools are created daily intended to improve care in the OR. Error reduction strategies using some of these newer technologies are as follows:

- Advances are plentiful in the field of electronic documentation. This not only benefits the patient by timely and institution-wide availability of information but also allows for data retrieval for clinical and administrative report cards.
- Limit repetitive tasks when possible. Radiofrequency identification technology, for example, is an emerging technology that offers new solutions for time-consuming tasks, such as sponge and instrument counts.
- Investigate bar code technology for use with implants, medications, and supplies to facilitate documentation and tracking.

ENVIRONMENT

Human factors science requires that the physical environment be considered to balance the work

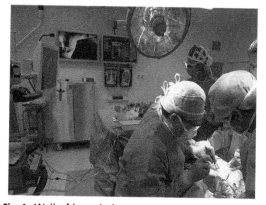

Fig. 4. Wall of knowledge.

system. Interaction among all components of the work system involves the environment, yet in health care, space constraints, outdated work areas, and inefficient planning can overcome any efforts to balance the system. With the increase in outpatient surgeries, technology, and concern regarding the conservation of resources, the physical environment is demanding attention. This presents an invaluable opportunity to bring human factor concepts to the OR.

One of the challenges in OR design and construction is to provide an efficient and safe environment for patients and staff. Standardization is the mainstay of error reduction strategies and should be considered in the design of the environment. During the design phase of a new 21-suite OR platform, Memorial Sloan Kettering Cancer Center developed principles to guide the design (**Fig. 5**). These principles were based on expert consultation and experience of the design team and were agreed upon by the executive committee. One of these guiding principles, "Promote familiarly and utility in room design though 95% similarity," addressed this notion of standardization. Just as agreeing on a process may make deviations from the norm more likely to be noted,[10] agreeing on a design of the OR may lead to surgical staff working more efficiently when stakes are high.

Vigilance refers to one's state of alertness and is particularly critical in risky conditions, such as in the OR. Promoting vigilance can be accomplished with the design of a nurses' workstation with full line of sight to the surgical field. At Memorial Sloan Kettering Cancer Center, the optimal height of the workstation was determined to be "transactional" height (42 inches) so that a nurse can sit or stand while accomplishing tasks. The controls for operating room lights, surgical equipment, and audiovisual integration were all designed to be within easy reach of nurses (**Fig. 6**). Sometimes consideration

of human factors, including the details of the environment, requires thinking out of the box. The openness to an "asymmetrical" orientation to the OR table, in which the OR table and light fixtures are not in the geographic center of the room, maximizes areas for sterile set-up and circulation. Regardless of the design, it is critical to get input from staff who work in the space. To the extent that it is financially and physically feasible, building a realistic mock up of the space to "play" in is an invaluable way to assess design plans.

Although the ideas presented for addressing the environment as a component of the system are resource-intensive, other strategies to consider might include the following:

- Lighting is important in the work environment. Multiple-zone fluorescent lights are useful for maximum control for maximally and minimally invasive procedures. Green lights can be considered for visualization by circulating staff and anesthesia during minimally invasive procedures.
- Temperature of the environment can affect the work balance. Design space outside the walls of the OR for electronic equipment. This approach allows for technical support from outside the procedure area, decreases the heat produced in the OR, and frees up valuable space around the patient.
- Planning flooring can save problems later. Consider hardness and cleanability and test several surfaces in a mock set-up if possible.
- Decrease number of steps necessary for staff when working in an environment. This goal can be accomplished by examining the workflow to identify locations for refuse, sharps, and laundry containers.

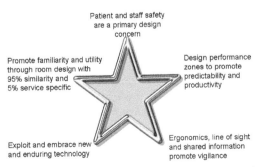

Fig. 5. Memorial Sloan Kettering cancer center operating room design principles.

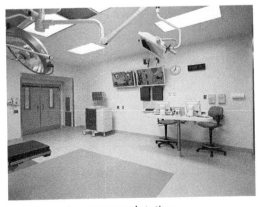

Fig. 6. Operating room workstation.

ORGANIZATION

The organizational context has implications for the work produced by the individual. To promote safety in the OR, emphasis on the importance of a safety culture throughout the organization is paramount. The value of a safety culture must be driven by senior leadership and diffuse to front-line staff. Programs that identify and involve patient safety champions or stars are useful in disseminating information to and from front-line staff. Cultivating this environment takes time, but several initiatives can facilitate the change.

The strongest predictor of a safety culture on the unit level is agreement with the statement "I am encouraged by my colleagues to report any patient safety concerns I may have."[26] Emphasis on reporting mechanisms can provide a rewarding start to building an organization conducive to patient safety. Although nurses traditionally have been the reporters of error,[27] responsibility should extend to include anyone involved in patient care. The reporting of errors should be simple, and well-designed computer-based programs are available to encourage reporting. For example, when Memorial Sloan Kettering Cancer Center instituted a computer-based reporting system, the reporting of actual events doubled. The organization also moved from reporting only incidents to reporting near misses, which was driven by use of a systems perspective.

Because near misses occur more often than errors, emphasis on near misses allows for the collection of more data, enabling organizations to most effectively identify weaknesses in the system that could lead to patient harm if not addressed. Reading groups, which consist of front-line and patient safety staff, review aggregate data for themes and process improvement opportunities that ultimately can serve the system in decreasing the number of "work arounds." Work arounds are first-order problem solving[28] and remove the immediate obstacle to getting work done but do nothing to change the probability of the event reoccurring. Whatever the mechanism of reporting chosen, feedback and nonpunitive discussions are critical in the development of trust in the system.

As in other industries, levels of teamwork in the OR correlate with the frequency of surgical errors.[29] Industries such as aviation have moved toward a culture that affords questioning by the crew and recognizes human limitations, however.[9] When attitudes toward teamwork and communication were examined among OR staff, however, nurses reported low levels of teamwork, whereas surgeons were in support of a hierarchy that functions to suppress the questioning of others' behavior or decisions.[9] Explicit opportunities for nurses and other staff must be made to encourage communication about concerns and specific patient issues. At Memorial Health System in Colorado Springs, 260 perioperative staff and physicians participated in 4 hours of focused human factor training. Before the training, the Safety Attitudes Questionnaire[30] was completed by more than 100 perioperative staff and physicians. This survey was repeated after the training and 1 year later

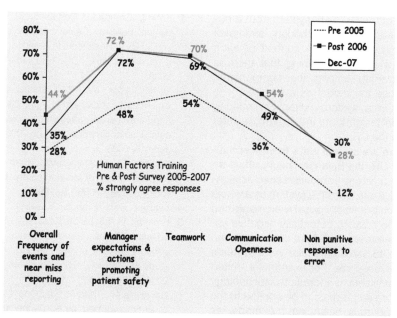

Fig. 7. Safety Attitudes Survey results.

after voluntary briefings had begun. The graph in **Fig. 7** represents five areas of significant improvement in regard to the perception of safety in the OR.

In addition to increasing reporting and facilitating teamwork, which are commitment-intensive strategies, organizations can cultivate a safer environment through the following means:

- Review policies pertaining to work schedules, corrective action, whistle blowing, and cultural competence with the Human Resources department.
- Shifting focus from the individual to the system not only gets to the real issues in the OR but also fosters job security through fairness.
- Consider institutional hiring practices. Balancing the work system may be made easier through careful selection of personnel. Southwest Airlines has a reputation for its "Hire for attitude, train for skill" philosophy.[31]
- Provide opportunities for professional development, such as a clinical ladder program and promotional opportunities. Participation in institutional committees and performance improvement projects not only increases perspective but also builds confidence and contentment with work.

SUMMARY

This article uses the Balance Theory to describe characteristics of the OR work system from a human factors perspective. Although examples have been provided within the context of each component, it is worth mentioning that there is considerable overlap among the components. The key is to use the model as a framework to guide thinking in a systems direction, offering new and different insights into the design of a safer work system in the OR.

Although there are several ways to conceptualize work in the OR, the Balance Theory offers an advantage in that no one particular aspect is highlighted. Instead, it examines the system as a whole to evaluate which potentially positive elements can be highlighted to balance potentially negative aspects.[15] This is especially helpful because it can be manipulated to serve particular work systems to best allocate resources. For example, if limited resources are available to address the technology component, more emphasis can be applied to the task component, thus balancing the model as a whole.

DIRECTIONS FOR FUTURE RESEARCH

The use of systems models, such as the Balance Theory, has not been readily tested within the context of health care systems. Although the use of strategies adopted in other systems can offer a unique and helpful approach, those lessons can only take the health care system so far. Likewise, the Balance Theory provides a framework for thought in the design of a safer OR; however, research is needed to explore the fit of the components to the OR system. Research designs that support testing the relationships between the elements as they pertain to the OR are necessary in the strategic development of interventions. This facilitates a trajectory of evidenced-based efforts to build a safer OR, which in time can be further tested to delineate the components that are predictors of a safe OR work system.

SUMMARY

"Human factors" refers to the application of knowledge of human strengths and limitations to the design of a work system. Valuable insight can be gleaned by borrowing from industrial applications of the human factors approach. The Balance Theory is one model through which the science of human factors can be brought to the OR. Through this model, elements of the work system in the OR are considered not as separate entities but as elements of a system that can be manipulated to provide safe care for patients.

REFERENCES

1. Kohn L, Corrigan J, Donaldson M, editors. To err is human: building a safer health system. Committee on Quality of Healthcare in America, Institute of Medicine. Washington, DC: National Academy Press; 2000.
2. HealthGrades, Inc. Third annual patient safety in American hospitals study April 2006. Available at: http://www.healthgrades.com/media/dms/pdf/patient safetyinamericanhospitalsstudy2006.pdf. Accessed June 16, 2008.
3. Christian CK, Gustafson MLZ, Roth EM, et al. A prospective study of patient safety in the operating room. Surgery 2006;139:159–73.
4. Leape L. Error in medicine. JAMA 1994;242:1851–7.
5. Brennan TA, Leape LL, Laird NM, et al. Incidence of adverse events and negligence in hospitalized patients: results of the Harvard medical practice study I. 1991. Quality and Safety in Health Care 2004;13(2):145–51.
6. Gawande AA, Thomas EJ, Zinner MJ, et al. Analysis of errors reported by surgeons at three teaching hospitals. Surgery 2003;133:614–21.

7. Rogers SO Jr, Gawande AA, Kwaan M, et al. Analysis of surgical errors in closed malpractice claims at 4 liability insurers. Surgery 2006;140:25–33.

8. Lingard L, Reznick R, Espin S, et al. Team communications in the operating room: talk patterns, sites of tension, and implications for novices. Academic Medicine 2002;77(3):232–7.

9. Sexton JB, Thomas EJ, Helmreich RL. Error, stress, and teamwork in medicine and aviation: cross sectional surveys. BMJ 2000;320(7237):745–9.

10. Wachter RM. Understanding patient safety. New York: McGraw Hill; 2008.

11. Weigmann DA, ElBardissi AW, Dearani JA, et al. Disruptions in surgical flow and their relationship to surgical errors: an exploratory investigation. Surgery 2007;142:658–65.

12. Yourstone SA, Smith HL. Managing system errors and failures in health care organizations: suggestions for practice and research. Health Care Management Review 2002;27:50–61.

13. Human Factors and Ergonomic Society. Available at: http://www.hfes.org/web/AboutHFES/about.html. Accessed June 11, 2008.

14. Smith MJ, Sainfort PC. A balance theory of job design for stress reduction. International Journal of Industrial Ergonomics 1989;4:67–79.

15. Carayon P, Smith MJ. Work organization and ergonomics. Applied Ergonomics 2000;31:649–62.

16. Mitler MM, Carkadon MA, Czeisler CA, et al. Catastrophes, sleep, and public policy: consensus report. Sleep 1988;11(1):100–9.

17. Gaba DM, Howardm SK. Patient safety: fatigue among clinicians and the safety of patients. N Engl J Med 2002;347:1249–55.

18. Committee on the Work Environment for Nurses and Patient Safety. Board on health care services: work environment of nurses. Available at: http://www.nap.edu/openbook/0309090679/html/1.html. Accessed June 18, 2008.

19. Rosekind M, Gander PH, Gregory KB, et al. Managing fatigue in operational settings. 2. An integrated approach. Hospital Topics 1997;75(3):31–5.

20. World Health Organization. Safe surgery saves lives. Available at: http://www.who.int/patientsafety/safesurgery/en/. AccessedJune 17, 2008.

21. Weick KE, Sutcliffe KM. Managing the unexpected. San Francisco: Jossey-Bass; 2001.

22. Battles JB, Keyes MA. Technology and patient safety: a two-edged sword. Biomedical Instrumentation & Technology 2002;36:84–8.

23. Vocera Communications Systems. Available at: http://www.vocera.com. Accessed July 8, 2008.

24. Kukla CD, Clemens EA, Morse RS. Designing effective systems: a tool approach. In: Adler P, Winogard T, editors. Usability: turning technology into tools. New York: Oxford University Press; 1992. p. 41–65.

25. Institute for Healthcare Improvement. Available at: http://www.ihi.org/IHI/Topics/Improvement/Improvement Methods/Tools/Flowchart.htm. Accessed on June 19,2008.

26. Perspectives on safetyIn conversation with Bryan Sexton. Available at: http://www.webmm.ahrq.gov/perspective.aspx?perspectiveID=34. Accessed on June 14,2008.

27. Lawton R, Parker D. Barriers to incident reporting in a healthcare system. Quality and Safety in Health Care 2002;11:15–8.

28. Edmonson AC. Learning from failure in health care: frequent opportunities, pervasive barriers. Quality and Safety in Health Care 2004;13(suppl 2):ii3–9.

29. Catchpole K, Mishra A, Handa A, et al. Teamwork and error in the operating room: analysis of skills and roles. Annals of Surgery 2008;247:699–706.

30. Sexton JB, Helmreich RL, Neilands TB, et al. The safety attitudes questionnaire: psychometric properties, benchmarking data, and emerging research. BMC Health Services Research 2006;6:44.

31. Carbonara P. Hire for attitude, train for skill. Available at: http://www.starttogether.org/docs/hiring.pdf. Accessed July 9, 2008.

Initiatives to Improve Patient Safety

Alecia Cooper, RN, MBA, CNOR

KEYWORDS

- Patient safety • Health care reform • Quality
- Preventable conditions

The United States faces a paradoxical health care situation. On the one hand, the level of care available, at least at certain facilities, is among the best in the world and many major medical breakthroughs and innovations occur in America. On the other hand, the American health care system is dysfunctional to the point that justifiable concerns are being raised about patient safety. About 15 million incidents of medical harm occur each year, averaging 40,000 such events a day.[1] In a large study (n = 44,000) of operations performed between 1977 and 1990, it was found that 5.4% of all surgical patients suffered complications, nearly half of which were attributable to error.[2] It has been found that 40% to 60% of surgical site infections are preventable and that antibiotics are overused, underused, misused, or used at the wrong time in 25% to 50% of all operations; the result is that as many as 13,027 perioperative deaths and 271,055 surgical complications could have been prevented.[3] A 2007 study found that hospital-acquired infections were associated with 99,000 deaths.[4] A well-known 1999 report stated that medical errors cost the American health care system between $17 and $29 billion.[5] The full extent of the problem is so vast that it has not yet been rigorously quantified.

One of the first challenges in addressing safety in American health care is that there might not be a uniform way to define "American health care." The *Dartmouth Atlas*, published by the Dartmouth Institute for Health Policy and Clinical Practice, found American health care is "remarkably uneven," with wide variations in the frequency of primary care, visits to medical specialists, hospitalization rates, and so on. These variations challenge popular assumptions about health care. At first glance, one is tempted to make a lot of assumptions that the *Dartmouth Atlas* subsequently deflates. For instance, facilities that spend more on care do not necessarily deliver better care. Conversely, some of the best care in the United States is provided by lower-cost providers. One might assume that different severities of illness are reflected in different spending levels, but that is also not the case. Therein lies the heart of the issue: high costs are more indicative of quality and safety issues than higher levels of care.[6]

In discussing why care costs much more at certain institutions, the *Dartmouth Atlas* attributes such variations to supply-sensitive care, in which the supply of a specific resource (such as number of specialists or hospital beds per capita) influences use rates. Although supply sensitivity influences health care spending, it does not necessarily deliver better care. Whether viewed from the patient's perspective (outcomes, technical quality, satisfaction with care provided) or the physician's viewpoint (quality of communication among physicians, continuity of care), higher spending is not associated with better care either for Medicare beneficiaries (in isolation) or for all patients who have serious illnesses cared for at major United States academic medical centers.

The relationship between cost and safety in American health care is complex. Medical errors carry a huge price tag for institutions, payers, and patients and their families. Yet the current American health care system is not set up for payers to exercise much control over the quality of care delivered.

Congress has called for fundamental reforms of the Centers for Medicare and Medicaid Services (CMS), moving it to a more proactive role from its previous role as "passive payer" that incentivizes health care consumption with no links back to quality or appropriateness. The original Medicare

Clinical and Marketing Services, Medline Industries, Inc., One Medline Place, Mundelein, IL 60060, USA
E-mail address: acooper@medline.com

Perioperative Nursing Clinics 3 (2008) 287–295
doi:10.1016/j.cpen.2008.08.006

program was designed to pay for care, as ordered, and to treat as inconsequential the quality of care. Medicare had no incentives (or even passive penalties) for such common-sense tactics as preventive medicine, withholding excessive care, or thorough patient education.[7] Under the Deficit Reduction Act Section 5001(b), CMS was authorized to develop a pay-for-performance or value-based purchasing (VBP) program for hospitals that would tie reimbursement to achievement of certain benchmarks or goals in quality and efficiency. VBP is considered a major paradigm shift in American health care. Although financial reform is no doubt needed, it is perhaps even more important to consider the role VBP could play in improving patient safety.

The Hospital VBP plan, to launch in 2009, will use measures, data infrastructure and validation steps, incentive structure, and public reporting. In setting up this program, CMS has identified that care ought to be safe, effective, efficient, patient-centered, timely, and equitable. The goal is first to quantify where hospitals are and then establish ways to measure improvement. Hospitals will be awarded a Total Performance Score, an aggregate of scores based on attaining certain benchmark levels and based on their own improvement over the prior year. This Total Performance Score translates into an incentive payment plan. The Hospital VBP plan has elevated patient safety to a key element of the Total Performance Score. Although safety is now tied to financial incentives, it may be of even more value that hospitals have been given ways to measure their levels of safety, to report safety data, to compare their data against established benchmarks, and to use safety scores as a way to identify specific areas for improvement. Of course, tying financial incentives to performance in a field as fraught with uncontrollable variables as health care can be a difficult leap of faith for hospital administration. Every health care provider knows that there are times that a clinical team can do everything right and still get a poor outcome.

The American Hospital Association (AHA) supports VBP, but advocates moving forward carefully and with deliberation to avoid the creation of convoluted or counterproductive incentive-based payment plans. In this regard, AHA set forth its guidelines to create a workable incentive program that includes focusing on improving quality (rather than cutting costs), incremental implementation, and using measures that are evidence-based, tested, feasible, and statistically sound, and that recognize differences in patient populations.[8] VBP initiatives are some of the most fundamental changes in American health

care in recent times, but other initiatives have already been used successfully to help address the safety issues in American hospitals. In 1996, the Institute of Medicine (IOM) of the National Academies in the United States launched a phased, multiyear initiative aimed at the large but important goal of improving the quality of health care in the Unite States. The first phase (1996–1999) reviewed medical literature to capture the scope of the problem, which can be summed up as the overuse, underuse, and misuse of available health care resources. In the second phase (1999–2001), the Committee on Quality of Health Care in American formulated metrics and a roadmap to help "cross the quality chasm" from what medical consensus determines to be sound health care practice versus what American patients actually receive. Now in its third phase, this initiative seeks to put its vision into practice by creating a "more patient-responsive health system."[9]

Initiatives to improve patient safety may seem fairly straightforward on the surface, but crafting them can be complicated. Such initiatives, both public and private, have been successful in accomplishing the goals the initiatives set for themselves and finding resonance with the clinical community. The result has been a spate of initiatives that has created a bit of its own confusion. In 2006, the AHA launched the AHA Quality Center to help hospital leaders keep abreast of the many new and effective measures in improving quality and patient safety.[10]

An effective initiative must involve two distinct entities and help restructure their interaction: health care services and health care systems.[11] The Agency for Healthcare Research and Quality (AHRQ) of the US Department of Health and Human Services formulated Ten Patient Safety Tips, which may be grouped into setting up quality programs at the hospital (continuous improvement, reporting systems, proper decision-making tools), creating an efficient working environment for clinicians (teamwork, limiting shifts, using appropriate-level staff, minimizing interruptions), and fundamental medical safety tips (infection prevention, proper use of chest tubes and urinary catheters, and so on). Part of AHRQ's role is to provide data necessary to formulate initiatives and assess quality levels. One such successful effort is the creation of the Consumer Assessment of Healthcare Providers and Systems patient questionnaire to evaluate the patient's perception of his or her care. Data pose a unique problem in patient safety initiatives. As the American health care market increasingly asks consumers to make important decisions in their own health care, the need for comprehensible patient safety data becomes urgent. Right now, hospitals follow no uniform national standards in what data they collect, how they collect them, and how these data are transmitted. Apples-to-apples comparisons can be impossible across systems. Variations in which data are collected and how they are collected can occur even among hospitals in the same system. For this reason, the National Voluntary Hospital Report Initiative, a public-private collaborative, launched a three-state pilot program in 2003 to standardize hospital data across all systems. The goal is to collect similar data in similar ways so that meaningful comparisons can be made across the continuum of care and among facilities.

Even today, the degree to which health care in the United States is consistent with basic quality standard is largely unknown, in part because quality studies tend to be highly focused and not indicative of overall care received by the average consumer.[12] It may thus be possible to obtain safety statistics for a specific procedure done in a specific time period at certain hospitals, but not broad safety statistics. This paucity of information contributes to the persistent belief in the United States that quality is not a serious national health care issue. In a comprehensive study, phone interviews with a random sampling of adults (n = 6712) in 12 American metropolitan areas evaluated performance on 439 indicators of quality of care for 30 acute and chronic conditions and for preventive care. Aggregate scores found that only about half (54.9%) of patients received recommended care.[13] What remains unknown is the real price tag for those patients who did not received recommended care—in financial terms and in human suffering and even loss of life.

The Institute for Healthcare Improvement (IHI) launched a groundbreaking initiative in 2004 with its aptly named 100,000 Lives Campaign, an initiative aimed at reducing deaths attributable to preventable medical errors. More than 3000 hospitals came together for an initial program credited with saving 122,000 lives in its first 18 months. Encouraged by national and grass-roots–level resonance, IHI launched its Five Million Lives campaign in 2006, aimed at preventing 5 million cases of medical harm over a 2-year period. More than 3800 facilities are enrolled in Five Million Lives, including more than 1500 rural hospitals (which have a special rural affinity group to address their unique needs). Building on the first six platforms of 100,000 Lives, the Five Million Lives Campaign added six more:

Deploy rapid-response teams at the first sign of patient decline.

Deliver reliable, evidence-based care for acute myocardial infarction to prevent death from heart attack.

Prevent adverse drug events by implementing medication reconciliation.

Prevent central line infections by implementing a series of interdependent, scientifically grounded steps.

Prevent surgical site infections by reliably delivering the correct perioperative antibiotics at the proper time.

Prevent ventilator-assisted pneumonia by implementing a series of interdependent, scientifically grounded steps.

Prevent harm from high-alert medications, starting with a focus on anticoagulants, sedatives, narcotics, and insulin.

Reduce surgical complications by reliably implementing all of the changes recommended by SCIP, the Surgical Care Improvement Project.

Prevent pressure ulcers by reliably using science-based guidelines for their prevention.

Reduce methicillin-resistant *Staphylococcus aureus* (MRSA) by reliably implementing scientifically proven infection control practices.

Deliver reliable, evidence-based care for congestive heart failure to prevent readmissions.

Actively work with hospital boards of directors, so that they can become more effective in accelerating organizational progress toward safe care.[14]

Participating hospitals pick at least one of the platforms to address, but are encouraged to tackle several. The 100,000 Lives and Five Million Lives initiatives demonstrate the role that a single hospital, acting independently, can play in improving patient safety. Although sweeping national programs are important, this sort of well-promoted initiative of individual facilities has also been effective.

The eighth platform of the Five Million Lives campaign refers to the Surgical Care Improvement Project (SCIP), a well-known initiative for surgical safety. SCIP's genesis began in 2002, when CMS and the CDC launched the Surgical Infection Prevention Project; findings from this project on preventable surgical site infections and inappropriate use of antibiotics resulted in the creation of SCIP, a suite of national initiatives aimed at improving the care of Medicare patients receiving surgery. The original goal of SCIP was to reduce preventable surgical morbidity and mortality by 25% by 2010. Using outcome, process, and test measures, SCIP commenced with a three-state pilot program (Ohio, Oklahoma, Kentucky) and deploying four modules of preventable complications:

Surgical infection prevention
Cardiovascular complication prevention
Venous thromboembolism prevention
Respiratory complication prevention[3]

Although such national-level initiatives seem lofty and academic, they can boil down to some practical solutions. For example, evidence-based guidelines have shown that delivering antibiotics to a surgical patient within 1 hour before the first incision can significantly reduce surgical site infections. The National Nosocomial Infections Surveillance system of the Centers for Disease Control and Prevention (CDC) have found that rigorous implementation of this guideline alone reduced surgical site infections up to 44%, with other organizations reporting similar results.[15] Simple and low-cost preventive measures often result in documentable quality improvements.

About 2 million adverse events involving drugs occur each year, owing to such causes as prescribing error, improper product selection or use, known side effects, or some yet-to-be identified problem. These adverse drug events account for approximately 100,000 deaths a year.[16] Out of this knowledge, the science of safety has emerged, helping us to grapple with the dilemma of modern health care, namely the trade-off between access and safety.[17] For example, assume several adverse events prompt the US Food and Drug Administration (FDA) to remove a drug from the market. What about the many patients who could have benefited from that drug? Taking the drug off the market will prevent some adverse events (safety), but at what cost to the patients who benefit from the drug and tolerate it well (access)?

In the United States, the FDA determines in a premarket phase whether a drug's benefits outweigh its associated risks for the labeled use in the intended population. Despite being one of the most rigorous approval processes in the world, the FDA system simply cannot uncover every possible safety problem. In most cases, early clinical trials are not large enough, diverse enough, or long enough to uncover all of the potential issues. Future studies and ongoing use often turn up rare, serious adverse events that may only occur with long-term use or in specific population subgroups or in combination with other treatments. New information about drug safety is often obtained after the drug has been on the market for a while.

The FDA handles this through so-called postmarket surveillance programs, which study adverse events reported for commercially available drugs. Postmarket surveillance relies on voluntary reporting from clinicians, facilities, and hospitals to manufacturers, who in turn are required by law to report adverse events to the FDA. Although manufacturers are generally compliant in the process, the system is inherently reactive in that it relies on voluntary reports from many people who may be unaware of the vital importance of reporting postmarket adverse events. Postmarket surveillance thus provides the FDA with, at best, sketchy information on how products actually perform in real-world clinical situations.

In 2007, the Sentinel Initiative was created as part of the FDA Amendments Act. It allows the use of Medicare data from CMS to help fuel the postmarket surveillance process. Relying on public-private partnerships, the Sentinel Initiative uses current electronic data to determine how prescription drugs are affecting patients. The Sentinel Initiative will develop a new electronic system to enable the FDA to query a broad array of information to identify postmarket adverse events. A CMS final regulation makes it possible for federal agencies, states, and academic researchers to use claims data from the Medicare prescription drug program (Part D) for public health and safety research, quality initiatives, care coordination, and other research and analysis.[18] The objective of the Sentinel Initiative is to launch the Sentinel System, a national, integrated electronic system for monitoring medical procedure safety. This effort is a phased long-term initiative with pilot programs now underway. Its goal is to allow data mining and research activities across multiple data systems while protecting patient privacy.

Other FDA initiatives for patient safety include MedSun, the Medical Product Safety Network, launched in 2002 by the Center for Devices and Radiological Health to help identify, understand, and solve similar problems with medical devices. More than 350 health care facilities, primarily hospitals, participate, and there are sub-networks, such as KidNet (for pediatric and neonatal ICUs) and HeartNet (from electrophysiology laboratories), to capture specific data.

Like many recent quality initiatives, the Sentinel System relies on electronic health care data. President George Bush set forth a goal that most Americans should have an interoperable electronic health record by the year 2014. Related technologies, such as e-prescribing and electronic decision support tools, will help improve risk management systems, better protect the public, and potentially reduce health care costs.[17]

Previous postmarket surveillance systems relied on paper data, which meant that it could take years for patterns of adverse events to emerge from reports. It is hoped that electronic surveillance will allow problems to percolate to agency and clinical awareness rapidly.

The Sentinel System seeks to build on existing electronic infrastructure rather than build new systems from scratch, so as much as possible data sources will be managed and maintained by their owners. Working with the Nationwide Health Information Network, the Sentinel System will integrate systems to allow for queries of multiple data sources. Part of the Sentinel Initiative involves standardizing data, creating user-friendly interfaces to input and access data, and formulating standard terminology for use in electronic records. One of its several goals is transparency, in that protocols, data, and results should be made available to consumers.

The goal of allowing consumers better insight into hospital safety and performance is not a new one. With many Americans charged by their health care insurance, employers, and even health care providers to make more of their own decisions about health care, the American public rightly demands—and requires—more information. Yet few hospitals offer the degree of data transparency consumers need. In 2002, the AHA launched the Hospital Quality Alliance (HQA) to promote such transparency and to make reliable, credible, useful information on hospital quality available to the public. Joined by various prestigious national organizations (American Association of Retired Persons, the AFL-CIO, Blue Cross Blue Shield Association [BCBSA], and others), the originally voluntary alliance was aimed at making safety data available to consumers. Congress soon linked submission of HQA-requested data to receipt of the full Medicare market-basket update for hospital inpatient payment. Data are available to the public at HQA's Web site (hospitalcompare.hhs.gov). The success of the HQA initiative is clearly evident in its year-over-year growth. The role of standardized, transparent, coherent data cannot be overemphasized.

The burden of record-keeping falls to the hospitals, however, who often must add staff (or take staff away from patient care) to manage the time-consuming tasks of data collection and reporting. At present, hospitals face multiple requests for data (often similar versions of the same data) from insurers, employer groups, accreditation organizations, and government agencies. For that reason, HQA strongly advocates that data on quality be reported once to HQA in one format, which will save time,

streamline reporting, help standardize data, and bolster the value of HQA's transparency initiative. Meanwhile, the HQA continues to identify key areas of quality that can be measured and reported. On the docket are infection prevention, surgical care, pediatric care, and care for patients who have chronic conditions. Efficiency data will also be collected. These data may become the foundation on which CMS bases future pay-for-performance programs, an action supported by the AHA.[10]

After October 1, 2007, Inpatient Prospective Payment System hospitals were required to submit data on their claims for payment indicating whether diagnoses were present on admission (POA). After October 1, 2008, CMS cannot assign a case to a higher diagnosis-related group based on the occurrence of one of the selected conditions (see list below) if that condition was acquired during hospitalization. All of the conditions listed are ones for which guidelines and interventions exist and that are deemed to be reasonably preventable. The 2008 conditions are:

> Foreign object retained after surgery
> Air embolism
> Blood incompatibility
> Catheter-associated urinary tract infection
> Vascular catheter-associated infection
> Surgical site infection—mediastinitis after coronary artery bypass graft, certain orthopedic surgeries, and bariatric surgeries
> Pressure ulcer
> Falls (specific trauma codes)
> Deep vein thrombosis/pulmonary embolism following total knee/hip procedures
> Poor glycemic control

Conditions (which must be high cost, high volume, or both) under consideration for future lists include surgical site infections, ventilator-assisted pneumonia, and *Staphylococcus aureus* septicemia.[7] The POA criterion has caused some concern at the clinical level in that it requires new procedures to be mapped out and implemented, but it represents an important shift in institutional thinking away from passive payment for health care consumption toward incentivizing preventive care, a principle most clinicians heartily endorse.

The National Quality Federation (NQF) set forth a list of Serious Reportable Adverse Events in 2002 that has since been nicknamed "never events" because not only are these errors preventable, they should never occur. Never events are unambiguous, indicative of a problem in the facility's safety system, and important for public accountability. Of the 28 never events, those involving surgery include: surgery on wrong body part, surgery on wrong patient, wrong surgery on patient, foreign object left in patient, postoperative death in normal-health patient, and implantation of wrong egg. Recent proposals suggest that payers may opt not to pay for never events. A few states have started requirements that never events be reported. One such state, Minnesota, averages about 100 such event reports a year.[19] (Statistics on never events are lacking in that reporting for most facilities is discretionary and usually not done. Based on Minnesota statistics, however, it is reasonable to assume that never events do occur, probably more frequently than most consumers realize.) Initiatives to combat never events have been set forth and NQF advocates that a root cause analysis be performed when a never event does occur.

Although many safety initiatives come from the government, medical organizations, and health care providers, some patient safety initiatives have been launched by payers. The BCBSA worked with the Harvard Medical School's Department of Health Care Policy and formulated seven initiatives under the banner "collaborating with providers" in the fourth quarter of 2007. Among these initiatives are:

  Hospital Patient Safety (Anthem Blue Cross and Blue Shield in Virginia), Quality-In-Sights Hospital Incentive Program (Q-HIP): Data from network hospitals are harvested and interpreted to provide feedback on key quality and safety metrics. Launched in 2003 in 16 network hospitals, it has since expanded to more than 60 facilities.

  Quality Physician Performance Program (Q-P3) was a spinoff of Q-HIP in the same participating facilities. It uses outcomes, processes, and quality measures to reward evidence-based medicine and best practices. Results showed complication rates for angioplasty and cardiac catheterization procedures decreased by 50% and 29%, respectively, over the prior year.

  Blue Cross Blue Shield of North Dakota launched a pilot collaborative initiative for diabetes management in 2005. Patients receive a suite of services including medication comprehension and self-management education. Compared with non-study patients, pilot study patients had lower costs for care, fewer emergency room visits and fewer inpatient admissions.

  Blue Cross Blue Shield of Massachusetts and CareFirst Blue Cross Blue Shield partnered in an initiative to move from paper to electronic prescriptions. This initiative involved a series of interventions across multiple stakeholders. One of the largest such initiatives in the nation, the program offered free e-prescribing devices, services, and software to up to 2500 providers. In its first 4 years, more than 10 million electronic prescriptions were generated through the collaborative. In 2006, e-prescriptions resulted in 15,000 drug interaction warnings and 7400 drug allergy warnings generated by the system and delivered to the prescribing physician as an alert message.

  Blue Cross Blue Shield of South Carolina launched the Web Precert initiative to shape hospital precertification into a streamlined online procedure. The organization reports that 46% of all precertification requests and inquires are now managed online, saving time and reducing long-distance phone calls.[20]

Premier has set up Perspective, a national clinical database of 500 of its network hospitals for benchmarking and quality improvement activities. Hospitals submit data to Perspective for analysis; in particular, outcome data are compared and areas for improvement identified. Related tools include Premier's Safety Surveillor, a web-based tool aimed at optimizing antimicrobial use to improve outcomes. It helps to manage a facility's infection control surveillance and combat hospital-acquired infections. Other tools for analyzing and measuring quality metrics are also available.[21]

The Joint Commission, which offers accreditation programs for hospitals, formulates National Patient Safety Goals by highlighting problematic areas in health care, reviewing the medical evidence, and then consulting with safety and medical experts to determine specific solutions. Insofar as possible, solutions are formulated to be both specific and system-wide. In June 2007, the Joint Commission's Board of Commissioners approved the 2008 National Patient Goals. The system allows a 1-year phase-in period that includes defined expectations for planning, development, and testing (by milestones) at 3, 6, and 9 months in 2008. Full implementation commences in January 2009. Among the National Patient Safety Goals are:

  Use of at least two patient identifiers before providing care, treatment or service
  Final verification procedure before any invasive procedure

Requirement that a "read-back" confirmation be performed when critical test results are communicated verbally (either by phone or face-to-face)

Standardization of abbreviations, acronyms, symbols, and dose designations

Standardization of "hand-off communication" process that allows the recipient opportunity to ask questions

Annual review of look-alike/sound-alike medications with action taken to prevent confusion among such drugs

Labeling of all medications and medication containers on and off the sterile field.[22]

The Association of Professionals in Infection Control and Epidemiology set forth its Vision 2012 to establish itself as the recognized leader in infection prevention and control by health care practitioners, policy makers, health care executives, and consumers. Among its many related initiatives are development of public reporting standards, playing a leadership role in emergency preparedness, and promoting zero tolerance for health care–associated infections.[23] Likewise, the Association of Perioperative Registered Nurses (AORN) has formulated several initiatives specifically to guide nursing professionals in the surgical suite. These programs include toolkits available to AORN members for deployment at the local level and include prevention and response to surgical fires, correct-site surgery, safe medication administration, "just culture" (for reporting and analyzing medical errors with the goal of improving patient safety, not hiding wrongdoing), communication in patient hand-off, and human factors in health care.[24]

One of the most original groups in initiatives for patient safety is the Leapfrog Group. In 1998, several employers with larger health care expenditures came together, finding themselves in the untenable position of spending vast sums for health care with no way to assess quality or compare providers. In 1999, the IOM issued a report suggesting that large employers should take steps for market reinforcement of patient safety standards. Calling its initiatives "leaps," the Leapfrog Group officially started in 2000.

Working with the NQF, the Leapfrog Group formulated Thirty Safe Practices for Better Healthcare, which offer initiatives in four areas and tie back to never events. The Leapfrog Group has an unusual initiative with regard to never events. Although such preventable errors should ideally never occur, if and when they do, the Leapfrog Group offers special recognition to those hospitals who report them and take other appropriate steps,

such as apologizing to the patient and family, performing a root case analysis, and waiving related charges. The theory is that those facilities that take aggressive steps to learn from such preventable errors will more rapidly approach the goal of zero never events.[19]

The Leapfrog Hospital Survey publishes reports on the efforts of more than 1300 hospitals to improve the efficiency of care and has set forth so-called "purchasing principles" by which Leapfrog members (employers who provide health care coverage) are expected to abide. Chief among these principles are educating and informing enrollees about the safety, quality, and affordability of health care, educating consumers in care comparisons, and rewarding providers for advances in safety, quality, and affordability. In 2006, the Leapfrog Group launched its inaugural reward program for hospitals, based on five measures of quality and efficiency. Measures are scored by participating hospitals and their data vendors. Hospitals rated "excellent" or "show improvement" along both dimensions qualify for rewards. This initial program is likely to be expanded with other steps. The Leapfrog Group is currently assessing ongoing pay-for-performance projects by other organizations to help in formulation of its own incentives.[25]

Perioperative care contributes significantly to patient outcomes and overall quality of surgical care; with about 30 million operations annually in the United States, it is a vast field with vast potential.[26] The National Voluntary Consensus Standards for Surgery and Anesthesia launched a perioperative care initiative endorsed by the NQF, funded by CMS, and encompassing 28 measures at the hospital level, 10 measures for ambulatory surgery, and 12 measures for clinicians.

The Hospital Quality Incentive Demonstration (HQID), a joint project between CMS and Premier, was the first national project designed to determine if economic incentives to hospitals would be effective in improving the quality of care to inpatients. Initially set up for 2 years, the project was extended 3 more years. Premier collects a set of more than 30 evidence-based clinical quality measures from more than 250 of its hospitals around the country. The quality measures were determined by HQID, which tracks process and outcome measures in five clinical areas: acute myocardial infarction, heart failure, coronary artery bypass graft (CABG), pneumonia, and hip and knee replacements.[27] Using CABG surgery as an example, the initiative reviews such measures as:

Aspirin prescribed at discharge
CABG using internal mammary artery

Prophylactic antibiotic received within 1 hour of surgical incision

Prophylactic antibiotic selection for surgery patients

Prophylactic antibiotic discontinued within 24 hours after surgery

Inpatient mortality rate

Postoperative hemorrhage or hematoma

Postoperative physiologic and metabolic derangement[28]

The HQID project was a test of one VBP model and serves as a guideline for the current CMS proposal before Congress, which ties payment to quality of care or specified outcomes.[29]

The upshot of this program is that it should help determine standard, meaningful measures for health care quality. Financial incentives are intended to help focus hospitals on benchmarking and measurement tools which, in turn, identify those areas needing improvement. This program represents an important milestone in the American health care system in that this is the first time that, on a national level, participating hospitals could qualify for additional Medicare payments based on performance in clearly defined clinical areas. More than 250 hospitals joined this program at its inception, agreeing to have their Medicare reimbursements tied directly to the quality of care they provide. Although this may seem like a small step, it indicates the fundamental change in thinking going on in many American hospitals. Clearly, patient safety, clinical outcomes, and reimbursement are being considered as interrelated items in ways that benefit not only payers and patients but also potentially hospitals and other health care providers.

Fundamental financial questions remain, however. What do quality and safety initiatives actually cost the health care system? For CMS, the HQID program is cost neutral in that incentive payments are offset by the reduction in cost of care. To be specific, in the third year of HQID, more than a million patients were treated in one of the five clinical areas of the initiative; participating hospitals improved overall quality by an average of 15.8%, more than 2500 lives were saved, and CMS ended up paying about $24 million in incentive payments. Other initiatives are hoped to be cost-saving programs. It is sometimes hard to define specific costs that such programs save, however. For example, if an initiative prevents a patient from developing a surgical site infection, what expense does that truly save the system? At best, cost savings can be captured as statistical extrapolations. Just as we may not truly appreciate the full scope of the problem of patient safety in our hospitals, we may not (at least in the short term) fully appreciate how much money these initiatives actually do save the system.

Although there is increasing political awareness and a lively public discussion about America's "broken" health care system, the main focus has always been universal health insurance or other equitable solutions to extending health care benefits to the entire population. Without diminishing the importance of this laudable goal, it is unrelated to the problems discussed here in variation in patient care, misuse of health care resources, and patient safety issues. Patient safety must rise to public and political awareness as an important and independent goal in and of itself in improving American health care. Patient safety initiatives at the national and local level, launched by public and private stakeholders, and embracing large goals or small steps, have proved to be remarkably effective in improving patient safety, reducing medical errors, and saving money. Such initiatives may begin with sweeping concerns, but they ultimately boil down to a list of tactics. Many of these tactical steps are simple, inexpensive, and not particularly difficult to implement. It is highly encouraging that the solutions to many knotty and seemingly overwhelming health care problems can actually be found in a series of small, specific steps crafted in the form of specific health care initiatives. Even more encouraging, these initiatives seem to find that reducing error, improving patient safety, and upgrading care across the nation is actually associated with lower health care costs.

REFERENCES

1. Protecting 5 million lives from harm. Brochure. Institute for healthcare improvement. Available at: http://www.ihi.org/ihi. Accessed June 11, 2008.

2. Kohn LT, Corrigan JM, Donaldson MS, editors. To err is human. Washington, DC: Institute of Medicine, National Academy Press; 2000.

3. Bratzler DW. Surgical infection prevention and surgical care improvement. Powerpoint. Available at: http://www.medqic.org/dcs.ContentServer?cid= 1136495755695&pagename=Medquic%2FOther Resource%2FOtherResourcesTemplate&c=Other Resource. Accessed June 17, 2008.

4. Klevens RM, Edwards JR, Richards CL, et al. Estimating health care associated infections and deaths in US hospitals. Public Health Rep 2007;122:160–5.

5. To err is human: building a safer health system. November 1999: Available at: http://www.iom.edu/ Object.File/Master/4/117/ToErr-8pager.pdf. Accessed June 17, 2008.

6. Wennberg JE, Fisher ES, Goodman DC, et al. Tracking the care of patients with severe chronic illness: The Dartmouth Atlas of Health Care 2008. Available at: http://www.dartmouthatlas.org. Accessed June 12, 2008.

7. Valuck TB. CMS' progress toward implementing value-based purchasing. Available at: http://www.ehcca.com/presentations/qualitycolloquiam6/valuck_la.ppt.

8. Improving quality and patient safety from American Hospital Association. Available at: http://www.aha.org/aha_app/issues/Quality-and-Patient-Safety/index.jsp. Accessed June 12, 2008.

9. Crossing the quality chasm: The IOM Health Care Quality Initiative. Available at: http://www.iom.edu/CMS/8089/aspx?printfriendly=true. Accessed June 3, 2008.

10. Improving quality and patient safety from American Hospital Association. Available at: http://www.aha.org/aha_app/issues/Quality-and-Patient-Safety/index.jsp. Accessed June 11, 2008.

11. Testimony on health care quality initiatives. Carolyn M. Clancy. AHRC before the Subcommittee on health of the house committee on ways and means. May 18, 2007. Agency for Healthcare Research and Quality, Rockville (MD). Available at: http://www.ahrq.gov/news/qtest319.htm. Accessed June 3, 2008.

12. McGlynn EA, Brook RH. Keeping quality on the policy agenda. Health Aff (Millwood) 2001;20(3):82–90.

13. McGlynn EA, Asch SM, Adams J, et al. The quality of health care delivered to adults in the United States. N Engl J Med 2003;348:2635–45.

14. Protecting five million lives from harm. Available at: http://www.ihi/org/ihi. Accessed June 11, 2008.

15. SCIP: a partnership for better care. Available at: http://www.medqic.org/dcs/ContentServer?cid=1136495755695&pagename=Medqic%2FOtherResource%2FOtherResourcesTemplate&c=OtherResource. Accessed June 17, 2008.

16. Lazarou J, Pomeranz BH, Corey PN. Incidence of adverse drug reactions in hospitalized patients: a meta-analysis of prospective studies. JAMA 1998;279:1200–5.

17. The sentinel initiative. Available at: http://www.fda.gov/oc/initiatives/advance/reporters/report0508.html. Accessed June 18, 2008.

18. Sentinel initiative launched to improve patient safety and quality of care. Press release. Available at: http://www.aami.org/news/2008/052708.fdacms.html. Accessed June 17, 2008.

19. FAQs on never events. Available at: http://www.leapfroggroup.org/for_hosptials/leapfrog_hospital_quality_and_safety_survey_copy/never_events. Accessed June 17, 2008.

20. Blue cross and blue shield initiatives recognized for increasing patient safety and efficiency. September 10, 2007 Press release. Available at: http://www.bcbs.com/news/bcbsa/collaborating-with-providers-2007.html. Accessed June 16, 2007

21. Infection control surveillance software-automated tools to fight the battle against hospital-acquired infections. Available at: http://www.premierinc.com/quality-safety/tools-services/performance-suite/infectioncontrol. Accessed June 18, 2008.

22. National Patient Safety Goals: facts about the 2008 National Patient Safety Goals. Available at: http://www.jointcommission.org/PatientSafety/NationalPatientSafetyGoals/08_nposg_facts.htm. Accessed June 18, 2008.

23. Vision 2012: the strategy. Available at: http://www.apic.org/AM/Template.cfm?Section=About_APIC&;Template=/CM/ContentDisplay.cfm&ContentFileID=4688. Accessed June 17, 2008.

24. Toolkit. Available at: http://www.aorn.org/PracticeResources/Toolkits/. Accessed June 17, 2008.

25. Hospital rewards program. Available at: http://www.leapfroggroup.org/for_hospitals/fh-incentives_and_rewards/hosp_rewards_prog. Accessed June 17, 2008.

26. National voluntary consensus standards for surgery and anesthesia: additional performance measures. Available at: http://www.qualityforum.org/projects/ongoing/surgicalfacilities/index.asp. Accessed June 18, 2008.

27. CMS/premier Hospital Quality Incentive Demonstration (HQID). Available at: http://www.premierinc.com/quality-safety/tools-services/p4p/hqi/index.jsp. Accessed June 16, 2008.

28. HQID methodology. Available at: http://www.premierinc.com/quality-safety/tools-services/p4p/hqi/methodology-yedar1-3.jsp. Accessed June 18, 2008.

29. Patient lives saved as performance continues to improve in CMS, Premier healthcare alliance pay-for-performance project. Press release dated June 17, 2008, Available at: http://www.premierinc.com/about/news/june08/p4pProject061708.jsp. Accessed June 18, 2008.

Competence, Nursing Practice, and Safe Patient Care

Linda Brazen, RN, MSN, CNOR*

KEYWORDS

- Perioperative nursing • Operating-room nursing
- Competence • Patient safety • Staff education

Competent, competence, competences, competency, competencies—all describe, but in no way define, the complexity of knowledge, skill, and ability that are the hallmarks of successful practice in any profession, including the nursing profession. Attempts to define it as a concept or to create a model of competence, or to measure it have been addressed for almost twenty years in the nursing education, staff development, and practice literature.

Yet, as much as the competence is relevant to all health care disciplines, consumers of health care, academic and clinical educators, student nurses, employers, and administrators, even a common understanding or consensus of what competence is or is not does not exist.[1] Implicitly though, competence is essential!

THE COMPETENCE CONTINUUM

Nursing faculty struggle to create curricula that provides content and teaching strategies to best prepare students with entry-level competencies. Health care facilities with registered nurse (RN) employees struggle with entry-level competence. Nursing administrators and directors struggle with obtaining the finances to support competence development, especially as it relates to safe patient care issues. Unit-based managers struggle to keep staff competent in light of constant increasing technologies. Clinical educators and staff-development specialists struggle to assess, validate, and maintain all the points along the continuum of competence: from the entry-level competences of graduate nurses, to the initial-competence of new hires, to the new- and ongoing-competence needs of staff. Distinguishing competence as it relates to intent and purpose provides a consensus about the requisite knowledge, skill, and ability inherent in professional clinical nursing practice.

Academic nursing education curriculum is designed to provide students with a baseline of knowledge and a real-time skill base that ensures they are a generically "safe" clinician upon graduation. Because of this intention, student nurses are prepared for success in earning a professional nursing license. There are issues in licensure that are beyond the scope of this article. Specific to competence, however, it may be argued that the licensure examination is a static test of knowledge for a dynamic practice; and does not and cannot provide an indication of accuracy in future performance. A more common idea is that an RN license provides a measurable criterion for schools and colleges of nursing and employers. The license is intended to insure that graduates from various types of nursing education programs will be equally successful.

In the workplace, employers use the RN license as a baseline indicator of an ability to do a job, competence not withstanding. However, nurses starting their career or those hired into a care setting that they have no experience in, are not always prepared to do the job. Employers who recognize this liability but use the recruit-to-retain strategy to hire candidates who value competence as a process that continues after their licensure, rather than an end product, are most successful. The quality, not the quantity, of new hires should

University of Colorado Hospital, Denver, CO, USA
* 12605 East 17th Avenue, Aurora, CO 80045.
E-mail address: linda.brazen@uch.edu

Perioperative Nursing Clinics 3 (2008) 297–303
doi:10.1016/j.cpen.2008.08.003

be considered because what RNs do with their basic education has become the indicator of success in this quantum age of nursing practice.[2] Currently, competence is not measured at the entry, but at the exit, of a nursing career.

The gap between knowledge gained through nursing education and its application to nursing practice is a conundrum when considering competence. Similarly, the gap between knowledge gained in the work setting and its implementation in practice is another challenge. Patients, as the recipients of nursing care, need competent RNs, and RNs need career competence. Competence is absolutely necessary, but is still without definition.

Continuing Competence

Competence is an issue in nursing education, for employers of nurses, and for nursing itself. There are regulatory agencies, professional organizations, accrediting bodies and, in the clinical practice arena, a certification process that creates challenges and opportunities for attaining and measuring RN competence. All of these entities consider and influence issues of competence. Since nursing is primarily a clinical, practice-based profession, the influence of these organizations reaches far into health care settings, traditionally the largest employers of RNs. The Joint Commission on Accreditation of Healthcare Organizations (JCAHO), the accrediting organization for health care facilities, requires employers to have programs in place that assess, maintain, and provide its employees with an ongoing process to maintain and gain competence.

Performance evaluation is a separate JCAHO requirement and process, and relates to issues of competence at the organizational and individual employee level. Recently the JCAHO added National Patient Safety Goals (NPSG) to their standards that measure, in part, the organization's and its employees' competence and performance. The JCAHO does not prescribe how to implement or to measure an organization's or an employee's performance. The expectation is that catastrophic errors and near-miss patient incidents in health care settings will never occur. The JCAHO added a *never event* list to the NPSG in 2006. It continues to review organizational performances, and update and create new standards as needed, in order to attain the goal of eliminating *never events* in patient care.[3]

The standards of practice set by specialty nursing organizations are used by health care facilities and RN employees to develop competencies. Most specialty nursing organizations publish evidence-based guidelines for practice, and support evidence in ongoing research. The results are then shared in professional journals. An additional set of guidelines and recommended practices, published with the standards of practice, are available from these organizations. These are used to develop work-place policies that support RN patient care competence. The Association of periOperative Registered Nurses (AORN) has published guidelines that support NPSGs.[4]

Other groups that also contribute to professional competence issues, literature, and practice settings are the credentialing bodies for each specialty practice. Research is lacking to demonstrate a link between certification exams and improved patient outcomes.[5] However, a number of credentialing organizations are exploring how to validate competence so that portability and reciprocity are options for certified RNs who change employers or move to another state. Continuing career competence, through certification by examination and by participation in competence and skills-based activities, would be profiled and transferable throughout their career and from employer to employer.

Organizational Competence

The goal of accreditation for the performance of a health care-facility is to decrease the competition to be all things to all consumers and to increase the ability to do what it does best. Historically, the word "competent" was used in accreditation manuals to indicate the quality of the organization by using quantitative measurements such as fewer undesirable patient outcomes compared to a neighboring organization. A patient could use to these determine the safety of the health care organization. A health care organization was considered competent if fewer patient risks were associated with it. In addition, it was implied that employees of a competent organization were themselves competent. In the scheme of accreditation, the mechanistic term "capacity" was often associated with a quantitative organizational measure and a perception of quality employees. Competent and accredited facilities demonstrated two performance measures: successful patient outcomes and the capacity to employ staff to provide such outcomes. Relative to the concept of competence, entry-level knowledge and skill combined with the RN license were considered equivalent to the knowledge and skill of the career-level competent RN in assigning roles and responsibilities. There was a plethora of health care, nursing education, and nursing practice literature published in this era about competency as it related to entry-into-practice issues; including the comprehensive work of Patricia Benner.[6]

In 1991, the word "competent" in the JCAHO manual was changed to "competence." This was a deliberate move on the part of the JCAHO Agenda for Change. The administrative and accreditation changes were designed to be less prescriptive and more process oriented. In turn, health care facilities were expected to be more process-oriented and to use competence as a criterion of performance. Instead of organizations attempting to provide all care to all consumers, each organization identified its competence according to what it did best; for example: organ transplant surgery, birthing center, or a specialization such as oncology. Since employee competence was a critical component of an organization's competence, the design of competence programs for employees was an indication of organizational performance. Employee competence programs included organizational expectations and identification of observable and measurable actions indicating individual performance. An employee who successfully demonstrated the combined performance of knowledge and skill had achieved competence. Implicit in the achievement was the expectation of continuing competence, which will be addressed in a later section of this article.

The terms "competent," "competence," and "competency" are often used interchangeably. Relative to accreditation standards, it may important to note that in addition to changing the word, the competence standard was moved from its original place in the nursing care standards section (1987–1991) to the staff education standards, where it remained until 1994. Then it was moved into the human resources article, where it remains as of this writing.

NATIONAL PATIENT SAFETY GOALS

Accreditation has evolved over the years, but what has remained constant is that it is a process, not a standardized or terminal point, along a continuum of patient care. Regardless of changes in the process of accreditation, the JCAHO sets the primary benchmark for the safety and quality of care provided to future and current consumers of health care. Patients, as the consummate consumers of services provided by health care organizations, have become actively engaged in determining the nature and quality of their own care and services. Through the years, the JCAHO has fostered and nurtured progressive and prospective process improvement initiatives in accredited health care organizations. This has been supported by consumers declaring that catastrophic errors and near-miss patient safety incidents are not acceptable. A representative group was invited to work with the JCAHO to explore and prioritize the elimination of untoward patient incidents. They reviewed current goals and suggested new goals, and recommended requirements, based on evidence and best practices, geared to prevent such incidents from occurring. These goals are presented in the NPSG section of the accreditation manual. Any organization, accredited or seeking accreditation, which offers health care-consumer care, treatments, and services relevant to NPSG is responsible for implementing the applicable requirements or effective alternatives. A term used in reference to the JCAHO Safe Patient Care Initiative is the "safety trilogy." Components of the safety trilogy are (1) trends in sentinel events, (2) preventative patient safety programs related to near-miss incidences, catastrophic errors, and *never events*, and (3) the NPSG.

ASSOCIATION OF PERIOPERATIVE REGISTERED NURSES

In general, NPSG are focused on system-wide solutions. As professional patient care providers, perioperative RNs, including those primarily in the intraoperative phase of patient care, are equally responsible for creating a culture of patient safety. Creating and maintaining a culture of patient safety is a measure of organizational and employee competence. The subsets of patient-safety culture include, but are not limited to:

A reporting culture, in which practice errors and near misses allow staff in the organization to learn from the experience.

A learning culture, in which gaining knowledge (ie, learning!) from experience is superseded by a willingness to implement major changes geared toward preventing any untoward incidences in the future.

A wary culture, in which members of all patient-care teams are continually alert for the unexpected.

A just culture, in which all members of a patient-care team are acutely aware of the distinction between acceptable and unacceptable behaviors, including appropriate and inappropriate behaviors.

Inherent in any patient safety culture is the mindset that all its employees share the values, attitudes, and beliefs of the organization; and that reporting without blaming is a strategy that supports and improves patient safety. To encourage employee buy in, an organization may use differing strategies, and technologies may be introduced to promote safe patient cultures. Learning to learn from knowledge, experience, and skill is the core of employee competence. If an entry-level employee's competence requirements are to learn unfamiliar or new technologies, to learn about communication expectations, and to learn that changing practice often reduces errors, then maintaining a "learning" process as a competence during the employee's tenure with the organization is achievable.

AMERICAN NURSES CREDENTIALING CENTER

The gap between education and practice will always be a challenge because it is created by a difference in competence as an outcome-based activity, not a terminal event. In nursing education, the outcome is to learn nursing. By achieving RN licensure, the graduate student nurse is generically "safe." In nursing practice, however, the outcomes are always and only patient-oriented. Since the practice role of competency from an educational perspective identifies and measures learning outcomes (also known as entry-level competencies), the result is that the competency of entry-level RNs have had to be met by employers through externships, internships, residency programs, orientations, in-services, and worksite continuing education programs.

Employers also had to meet the continuing, ongoing, and career competence of employed RNs. Often, this was achieved through certifications, portfolios, and progressive skill building to bridge performance expectations in the workplace. Clinical-based RNs have concerns about the quality of care they provide and the safety of their patients, and they want to work with competent peers. Knowing that a practicing RN is ready and able to provide care at the highest level of ability is also important to patients, colleagues in other health care disciplines, legislators, and organizations.[7] Accountability to oneself to be a competent peer is tantamount to being a safe care-giving professional. Everyday nursing practice takes place in dynamic health care systems that are bursting with new knowledge and skills to learn, and a multitude of decisions that must be made to keep patients safe.

As a practicing RN, it is a challenge to maintain competence and to demonstrate competence if employment changes. In an attempt to facilitate competence portability and competence reciprocity, the American Nurses Credentialing Center (ANCC) created Nursing Skills Competency Accreditation.[8,9] The program is designed as a voluntary process for health care facilities to provide educational or training activities that yield or validate a nursing skill or subset. The ANCC Commission on Accreditation validates that a provider meets established standards based on predetermined criteria. Unlike the ANCC program that accredits organizations for Magnet Status, accreditation is awarded to an individual educational activity that meets design criteria. The activity must have both a didactic and a skills-demonstration component, and requires validation and reliability. The program is a tool for employers and individual nurses to use to identify educational programs that are appropriately designed to validate nursing skills and skill sets. Employers and health care consumers would have confidence that an RN met competency requirements.[9]

COMPETENCY & CREDENTIALING INSTITUTE

The quality of certification in nursing practice is indicated by the number of certified RNs. The value of a health care facility employing certified RNs is that it receives the ANCC Magnet Status Accreditation. The Competency & Credentialing Institute (CCI) is the leader in credentialing the operating room (OR) nursing community, and has supported and facilitated a number of competency credentialing education programs since 1979.[10] Credentialing entails achieving success on a national examination. Competence entails maintaining credentials through participation in specific education activities which include but are not limited to ANCC-approved continuing education. In 2007, CCI convened the national Think Tank to explore how those in nursing can collaborate to develop a framework for continuing competence. As a number of definitions of competence were reviewed and themes emerged, a number of action items were identified for the nursing profession to consider when developing or implementing continuing competence programs and activities.[11] These themes included:

Competence is evolutionary; it is a process and an outcome.
Educational process needs reform; competency-driven learning and student self-awareness are critical.
Information literacy needs to be developed.
Knowledge is dynamic, evolutionary, and experiential; needing to know is not as important as needing to retain.
Social, public, health, and economic influences are dynamic factors in health care worker competence systems.

- Working and learning in multidisciplinary teams is an essential component for the delivery of safe patient care.
- Data management is crucial because the effective use of data can help determine what constitutes safe patient care and safe nursing practice.

COMPETENCE APPLICATIONS

Healthcare organizations can have the most competent RN staffs, but if the environment is not supportive of professional practice, safe practice for patients will fail. Infrastructure programs are important for entry- and career-level competence assessment, development, and maintenance. However, competence in relation to patient safety and patient outcomes may require innovative approaches such as developing the competence process after both patient safety and patient outcomes are established. Instead of using static policies as a guide for care practice, a competence in a specialty of nursing could be the catalyst for the RN to design, manage, and coordinate the patient's care according to the variables presented.[1] Or, a Synergy Model could optimize the nurse–patient relationship by matching the needs of the patient with the competencies of the RN, insuring a safe passage through the health care system for the patient.[12] Continuing a reverse mode of thought would mean that entry-level competence assessment, staff orientation, and all the other methods of staff education would also need to change. Fundamentally, the premise of the model is that patient characteristics drive nurses' competences.[7]

Gaps in knowledge, skill, and ability to provide safe journeys for patients as they transit through phases of care may be narrowing. In 2005, using a Robert Wood Johnson Foundation Grant, respected leaders from nursing education programs embarked on the Quality and Safety Education for Nurses (QSEN) Project.[13] The project's long-range goal is to reshape professional identity formation in nursing to include commitment to quality and safety competencies. To date, six specific quality and safety competencies for nursing have been identified and developed; and targets for the knowledge, skills, and attitudes to be developed in nursing pre-licensure programs have been proposed. The six core competences are (1) patient-centered care, (2) teamwork and collaboration, (3) evidence-based practice, (4) quality improvement, (5) safety, and (6) informatics. The second phase of QSEN includes partnering with representatives to discuss potential graduate education competencies, and working with 15 pilot schools that voluntarily committed to change their curricula toward incorporating quality and safety competencies. The QSEN Project is an academic response that may bridge the knowledge, skill, and ability gaps in competence for nursing students when they are hired into their first professional clinical position. The project is a model that, perhaps in combination with the myriad of new gradate programs created by a number of health care facilities to address the gap, may literally solve the issue of entry-level competence.

The other end of the nursing competence continuum concerns the gaps in knowledge, skill, and ability of practicing nurses. Career competence includes achievement and maintenance of specific competencies associated with an RN's area of expertise and practice setting.[14] As an RN, career core competence includes the abilities to think in action, have confidence and clarity in decision-making, and to retrieve information. In the depth and breadth of health care, education, and nursing literature over the years, multiple models, methods, and strategies have been utilized to control the competence continuum in work-place settings. Clinical nursing practice is desperate for a blueprint that assures achievement and maintenance of competences that will improve clinical nursing and provide patients with safe journeys through their health care experience. To date, what is conclusive is that, on the whole, we have a very poor understanding of our own ability to change health care worker behaviors.[15] Delivery of knowledge content has rarely embraced measuring the outcomes of learning (ie, competences). As a result, health care employers face the dual struggle of evaluating competency and managing the regulatory and accrediting challenges of patient safety. Measuring annual competence by evaluating RN clinical bedside skills does not guarantee that an RN possesses the actual knowledge, skill, and ability to care for patients, and to care for them in changing patient situations.

COMPETENCE, OPERATING ROOM NURSING PRACTICE, AND SAFE PATIENT CARE

Self-assessment is both a challenge and an opportunity when it comes to accountability. Society has conditioned people to believe that high self-esteem is more important than anything else. One unfortunate side effect is that people can come to view anything other than praise as a personal attack, or a sign they are not knowledgeable and talented. Self-assessment is a critical component of any professional's behavior, and competence is an ethical component. Self-assessment requires a person to examine and be accountable for their actions and competency. Ethically, if one's actions are parallel with expectations of society and regulatory, accrediting, and credentialing agencies, self-assessment is an opportunity to be accountable for one's own practice.

Safe patient care in OR care settings requires competence in OR nursing practice. At the core of that practice is the higher level practice concept of advocacy. As an OR RN, advocating for patients in need of operative procedures is to guard them against errors and to provide them with competent practices when they are at their most vulnerable. Efforts toward the goals of self-assessment, accountability, and competence are in place through mutual collaborative initiatives such as the Council on Surgical and Perioperative Safety[16] and JCAHO International Center for Patient Safety.[17]

Competence and accountability at a day-to-day level of practice are both a challenge and an opportunity. It has long been a challenge to assess intraoperative patient outcomes only associated with RN competence.[18] As indicators of what patients should expect from nursing care during surgical or other invasive procedures, the outcomes have never been intended to be only the result of a patient's time in the OR. Nonetheless, how the patient actually benefited as a result of an RN's advocacy has not been identified through the number of tasks and interventions performed and documented by the intraoperative RN during the patient's intraoperative experience.

The impact of emphasizing the RN's actions, rather than how the patient benefits from those actions, is unknown at this time. Instead of being fearful that unlicensed staff will encroach on an RN's practice, RNs in the OR setting can turn this perceived challenge and their tasks and interventions into an opportunity for a patient's safe journey. The opportunity at a day-to-day level is not found in asking who is responsible for the patient's safe journey, but realigning the question into a framework that through competence and accountability make all of us as professionals responsible. Under pressure from insurers, federal, and regulatory agencies, hospitals are starting to agree to not charge a patient who experiences a *never event*, because a *never event* should not have happened.[19]

The cost of treatment resulting from surgical objects left in a patient during surgery, patient falls, catheter-caused urinary tract infections, and pressure sores will no longer be reimbursed because these errors occurred during a hospital stay. The incentive for health care workers to be vigilant to competence, accountable for practice, and responsible for working in collaboration is clear. Building a culture of safety using high reliability principles is key to the future success of health care facilities as employers of professional RNs. To support these efforts, standardized practice strategies have been designed.[20,21] In the literature, evidence can be found that relates how systems and interactions between system components influence performance and patient safety.[22]

SUMMARY

There will always be health care consumers and there will always be a need to help them go safely through their health care experience. Patient outcomes that indicate achievement of safe patient care are needed for RNs. Their competence must be based on a reality of patient-focused phenomena and patient-focused outcomes. Traditional psychomotor approaches to skill acquisition and cognitive delivery methods for knowledge acquisition have not fostered changes in health care worker behaviors. Evidence based entry-level and career competence strategies need to incorporate abilities including, but not limited to, attention to patient safety and cue recognition of emerging patient crisis. There is also a need for support from the organizational level for human and fiscal resources to design and develop relevant content.[23] Optimal patient care depends on the best match between a patient needs, the nurse's advocacy practice, and nursing competence. When entry-level through career-level competence is finally defined, philosophical and operational changes in clinical staff education activities such as orientation, professional and staff development, in-service training, continuing education, and management development will need to occur.

REFERENCES

1. Tilley D. Competency in nursing: a concept analysis. J Contin Educ Nurs 2008;39(2):58–64.
2. Porter-O'Grady T. A glimpse over the horizon: a new future for nursing practice. In: A continuing education program designed specifically for the University of Colorado in Denver, College of Nursing. Denver (CO): Office of Professional Development and Extended Studies (OPDES); 2008.
3. Catalano K. Joint Commission and National Patient Safety Goals: Update for 2008. Presentation at the Association of periOperative Nurses Congress. Joint Commission on Accreditation of Healthcare Organizations. 1991 Accreditation Manual for Hospitals, Vol. 1: Standards 1990. Oakbrook Terrace, IL.

4. Association of PeriOperative Registered Nurses. Perioperative standards and recommended practices 2008. Denver (CO).

5. Wittaker S, Smolenski M, Carson W. Assuring continued competence: policy questions and approaches. How should a profession respond?. Available at: www.nursingworld.org/ojin. Accessed January 4, 2008. Joint commission on accreditation of healthcare organizations. Comprehensive accreditation manual for hospitals. Oakbrook Terrace, IL.

6. Benner P. From novice to expert: excellence and power in clinical nursing practice. Menlo Park (CA): Addison-Wesley Publishing Company; 2008.

7. Pacini CM. Synergy: a framework for leadership development and transformation. Crit Care Nurs Clin North Am 2005;17:113–9.

8. Overview of ANCC: Nursing Skills Competency Program: a new kind of nursing accreditation. Available at: www.nursecredentialing.org. Accessed July 7, 2008.

9. Yoder-Wise P. Continuing competence: one state's efforts. J Contin Educ Nurs 2008;39(2). 51.

10. Competency and credentialing institute. Available at: www.cc-institute.org/abus.aspx. Accessed July 7, 2008.

11. The CCI Continued Competence Forum: from pieces to policy. Available at: www.cc-institute.org/tt07. Accessed March 11, 2008.

12. Kerfoot KM, Cox M. The synergy model: the ultimate mentoring model. Crit Care Nurs Clin North Am 2005;17:109–12.

13. QSEN: Quality and Safety Education for Nurses: overview. Available at: http://qsen.org/competency domains. Accessed June 11, 2008.

14. Allen P, Lauchner K, Bridges RA, et al. Evaluating continuing competence: a challenge for nursing. J Contin Educ Nurs 2008;39(2):81.

15. Zero tolerance for infections: a winning strategy. Available at: www.infectioncontroltoday.com. Accessed May 11, 2008.

16. Banschback SK. Mutual accountability for the common goal of patient safety. AORN J 2008;88(1):11–3.

17. Joint Commission International Center for Patient Safety. Available at: www.jcipatientsafety.org. Accessed June 11, 2008.

18. Kleinbeck S, McKennet M. Challenges of measuring intraoperative patient outcomes. AORN J 2000; 72(5):845–53.

19. The basics: hospitals won't get to bill for errors. Available at: http://www.articles.moneycentral.msn.com/Insurance/InsureYourHealth. Accessed March 7, 2008.

20. Performance of correct procedure at correct body site: patient safety solutions. Available at: www.jcipatientsafety.org. Accessed June 11, 2008.

21. Patient safety practices: an online resource for improving patient safety. Available at: www.jcipatientsafety.org/22784. Accessed June 11, 2008.

22. Christian CK, Gustafson ML, Roth EM, et al. A prospective study of patient safety in the operating room. Surgery 2006;139(2):159–73.

23. Rapala K. Mentoring staff members as patient safety leaders: The Clarian Safe Passage Program. Crit Care Nurs Clin North Am 2005;17:121–6.

A Focused Review: Perioperative Safe Medication Use

Linda J. Wanzer, Col (Ret), MSN, RN, CNOR[a],*,
Rodney W. Hicks, PhD, MSN, MPA, FNP-BC, FAANP[b],
Bradlee Goeckner, LCDR, MSN, RN, CNOR[c],
Lisa Cole, MAJ, MSN, RN, CNOR[d]

KEYWORDS

- Medication errors • Perioperative care
- Perioperative nursing • Anesthesia • Surgery
- Ambulatory surgery • Same-day surgery
- Outpatient surgery • Medication system
- Drug administration • Operating room • MEDMARX

In 1859, Florence Nightingale wrote in *Notes on Hospitals*, "It may seem a strange principle to enunciate as the first requirement in a hospital that it should do the sick no harm."[1] This tenet had already been the basis for physicians, given the centuries-old standard of "first and foremost, do no harm." Yet, there remains public concern among patients who enter the health care system, and rightly so. Within the last decade, the Institute of Medicine (IOM) brought renewed attention to this hallowed tenant through its seminal report, *To Err Is Human: Building a Safer Health System*, when it asserted that up to 98,000 deaths occurred annually as the result of medical errors.[2] Citing data that health care institutions had caused harm and death,[2] the IOM went further in describing the health care system of the twenty-first century. In the newer model of patient safety, through the avoidance of iatrogenic injury, safety would be the new and minimally accepted standard of care.[3] Because of these reports, patient safety has become a mantra now espoused by all within health care.

Safe medication use has always been but just one important aspect of patient safety. Violations of safe medication principles, policies, and processes and the resultant medication errors now serve as the markers of evidence for warranted concern. Such markers gain worldwide attention through headline stories that reflect personal tragedies of countless victims. Although the full extent of how many medication errors occur is unknown, there are indicators of the pervasiveness of such system failures and, as such, reflect poorly on the world's most advanced health care system. The IOM claimed that up to 7000 deaths were directly attributable to medication errors.[2] Other investigators have estimated that errors can affect 20% of all routinely administered medications doses.[4] Researchers from the Food and Drug Administration investigated the agency's medication error database, the Adverse Event Reporting System, and found that 10% of the reported errors over a 6-year period resulted in fatality.[5] Still, other investigators have claimed that up to 9% of all hospital

The views expressed are those of the authors and do not reflect the official policy or position of the Uniformed Services University of the Health Sciences, the Department of the Defense, or the United States Government.
[a] Graduate School of Nursing, Uniformed Services University of the Health Sciences, 4301 Jones Bridge Road, Bethesda, MD 20814, USA
[b] Anita Thigpen Perry School of Nursing, Texas Tech University Health Sciences Center, 3601 Fourth, Mail Stop 6264, Lubbock, TX 79430-6264, USA
[c] Perioperative Department, Naval Medical Center San Diego, 34800 Bob Wilson Drive, San Diego, CA 92134-5000, USA
[d] 96th Medical Group, Eglin USAF Regional Hospital, 307 Boatner Road, Eglin Air Force Base, FL 32542, USA
* Corresponding author. 7600 Augustine Way, Gaithersburg, MD 20879.
E-mail address: lwanzer@usuhs.mil (L.J. Wanzer).

admissions result from medication errors.[6] In fact, medication errors, as of December 31, 2007, were the fourth leading reported sentinel event in hospitals across the United States according to the sentinel event statistics reported by the Joint Commission. Given that all medication errors are preventable,[7] it is no wonder that safe medication use became a focal point in numerous initiatives aimed at reducing the burden of iatrogenic injuries.

Since the release of *To Err Is Human*, great strides have been made to better understand the complexity of the health care system and how that complexity affects patient safety.[8] In turn, this understanding has guided the development of or revisions to professional guidelines,[9] national and international campaign initiatives focused on safety,[10] and state and federally mandated laws.[11] Many of these activities have influenced safe medication practices to help guide processes that move the health care delivery system to one that ensures that patient safety is the standard of care.[13]

The purpose of this article is to expand the perioperative team's knowledge about current safe medication practices. To accomplish this broad objective, the authors (1) build the knowledge base using definitions from a national taxonomy and a leading patient safety organization, (2) present findings from multiple sources that represent some of the known failure points that reflect the state of the science, and (3) propose and identify solutions to address the failure points. This discussion should allow perioperative clinicians to gain an appreciation of how the complex system within the perioperative environment predisposes otherwise competent practitioners to medication error involvement.

NATIONALLY AND INTERNATIONALLY RECOGNIZED CONCEPTS ASSOCIATED WITH ERRORS
The Value of Medication Error Reporting

Event reporting systems can be powerful tools to build knowledge when the findings are used to improve systems and educate providers.[12] The intent behind such systems is to collate and analyze the risks associated with related activities to propose remedial and preventive actions.[13] A reporting system is inclusive of multiple components: empiric and theoretic models, a variety of tools built from domain content, and analysis by domain experts.[14]

Even before *To Err Is Human* was published, *United States Pharmacopeia* (USP) had suggested significant patient safety initiatives drawn from the evidence of two national medication error reporting programs: the USP Institute for Safe Medication Practices Medication Errors Reporting Program and MEDMARX. The Medication Errors Reporting Program is a voluntary program open to all clinicians in all settings. This database, which is operated in cooperation with the Institute for Safe Medication Practices, collects information and provides data to regulatory agencies, professional organizations, and the pharmaceutical industry in an effort to educate about preventing future adverse drug events. MEDMARX, launched in 1998, is an Internet-accessible, anonymous medication error database used by hospitals and health systems and is available through an annual subscription service. MEDMARX provides subscribers with an opportunity to track adverse medication events within the facility, review errors reported by other facilities in the database, conduct comparisons between facilities, and examine quality improvement initiatives that other facilities have implemented in response to medication errors.[15] Although the facilities that report to MEDMARX currently comprise less than 10% of all United States hospitals and health care systems, USP has amassed the largest repository of medication error data currently available in the world, with more than 1.25 million case reports from more than 770 facilities. It is important to note that the number of case reports represents only those that have been voluntarily reported to MEDMARX.

When discussing the concept of reporting, it is important to recognize that two aspects occur: errors are reported and errors are not reported. Errors not reported can be further segmented into those intentionally not reported or those that are not detected. The Iceberg Model is an excellent representation of this phenomenon. Researchers[4,16,17] have studied the relationship of detected versus reported errors, and their findings indicate wide variances seen between what is reported (the tip above the water line) and what is undetected and remains unreported (the below the water ice mass). Furthermore, extending the analogy and comparing reporting versus not reporting, the mass that remains "underwater" represents lost opportunities to learn from mistakes that could be used to improve health care systems.

Leape[13] identified seven characteristics of successful reporting systems based on published expert opinions. The characteristics are (1) nonpunitive (free of fear of retaliation); (2) confidential (deidentified patient, reporter, and institutional information); (3) independent (analysis is done by an organization without power to punish); (4) expert analysis (content experts); (5) timely (prompt); (6) responsive (dissemination of results); and (7) systems oriented (focused on changes in systems and processes rather than on individual performances). Applying these characteristics to perioperative conditions (including errors) yields richness within practice to advance the profession.

National Coordinating Council for Medication Error Reporting and Prevention

Before discussing medication errors, the common languages used to report, analyze, and discuss medication errors and the medication use process (MUP) must be understood. Our understanding today of medication errors can be attributed to several sources, including early work done by the National Coordinating Council for Medication Error Reporting and Prevention (NCC MERP). Formed in July 1995 from 22 different constituent-based organizations,[1] NCC MERP and its members cooperatively addressed the multidisciplinary causes of medication errors to promote safe medication use.[18] NCC MERP produced the nation's first comprehensive taxonomy for studying medication errors and established the nationally recognized definition of a medication error. Accordingly,

*A medication error is any **preventable** event that may cause or lead to inappropriate medication use or patient harm while the medication is in the control of the health care professional, patient, or consumer. Such events may be related to professional practice, health care products, procedures, and systems, including prescribing; order communication; product labeling, packaging, and nomenclature; compounding; dispensing; distribution; administration; education; monitoring; and use.[7]*

The value of any taxonomy lies in its usefulness to provide a standard approach to record, interpret, and track phenomena. The NCC MERP Taxonomy of Medication Errors is the most useful tool known to evaluate medication error studies, given that it encompasses all disciplines involved in safe medication use.

Medication Error Severity

NCC MERP also created the Index for Categorizing Medication Errors to determine the outcome or effect of the medication error on the patient. The index contained four major subscales: potential for error (category A); actual error that did not reach the patient (category B); actual error that reached the patient but did not result in harm (category C or D); and actual error that reached the patient and resulted in harm (category E, F, G, H, or I). The reliability of this scale ($\kappa = 0.60$) was established in 2007 through a group of researchers at The Ohio State University.[19]

Medication Use Process

The MUP is a systems approach that defines the typical manner in which medications move through an institution in terms of prescribing, dispensing, and administering to patients.[20] According to USP, each step or point in the MUP is referred to as a node.[15] Each node represents domains of professional responsibilities, including the corresponding series of checks and balances and professional judgments that seek to ensure safe medication use. **Table 1** lists the nodes of the MUP and the corresponding definitions.

Nursing school curriculums and nursing practice have historically drawn heavily on one safe medication practice known as the "five rights," which intended to ensure that the right patient received the right dose of the right drug at the right time and by the right route. As a guiding practice, nurses have used this practice extensively. Furthermore, the practice has served as the legal standard for safe practice, because satisfying each of the "rights" offered maximum protection against medication errors. Yet, this practice is not fool proof, given that the national medication error reporting program MEDMARX contains data suggesting that one third of the reported medication errors that transpired between 2002 and 2006 occurred during medication administration.[21]

The continued prevalence of medication errors during drug administration indicates that the practice of five rights alone is not adequate to keep - patients safe from medication errors. So found the Illinois Court of Appeals when it rendered its decision that hospitals were responsible for the negligence of nurses performing physicians' orders by giving medications that were clearly contraindicated for the patient.[22] In this particular case, there was an underlying "assumption" that there was correct execution of tasks in all of the preceding steps within the MUP that ultimately proved to be inaccurate. Directly resulting from this case, two additional rights (the right indication and the right documentation) now embellish the standard for using medications safely. Furthermore, this case set legal precedence that, in effect, raised the bar by indicating that the five rights should not be the sole "safety net" for medication administration. Rather, undertaking

---

[1]A delegate from the American Nurses Association (Washington, DC) represents professional nursing.

Table 1
The medication use process

Node	Definition
Procuring	The formal action of how organizations obtain products
Prescribing	The action of a legitimate prescriber to issue a medication order
Transcribing	Anything that involves or is related to the act of transcribing an order by someone other than the prescriber for order processing
Dispensing	A phase that begins with a pharmacist's assessment of a medication order and continues to the point of releasing the product for use by another health care professional
Administering	A phase in the MUP in which the drug product and the patient interface
Monitoring	The phase that involves evaluating the patient's physical, emotional, or psychologic response to the medication and then recording such findings

From Hicks RW, Becker SC, Cousins DD, editors. MEDMARX data report. A report on the relationship of drug names and medication errors in response to the Institute of Medicine's call for action. Rockville (MD): Center for the Advancement of Patient Safety, US Pharmacopeia; 2008. p. 159–62; with permission.

a review of all steps of the entire MUP before administering a medication should be required to protect the patient.

Case scenario

A surgeon unknowingly writes an order for regular insulin, 10 U, in the wrong patient's chart. The patient for whom the surgeon is writing the insulin order is not diabetic. A pharmacist fills the order and sends the medication to the operating room (OR). The pharmacist perpetuates the error by labeling the medication with the name of the patient on the order sheet. A perioperative nurse, with faulty information, confirms the five rights and administers the insulin, further perpetuating the original error, and this patient becomes a victim of a medication error. The five rights failed as a safety net for the nurse and the patient in this case scenario. In addition, had this been a real case, based on the appellate court ruling from Illinois, the organization would have been liable in giving the patient the insulin because the patient was not diabetic. This case scenario demonstrates how the addition of the two new rights (the right indication and the right documentation) to the current five rights could add a new dimension to the safety net for medication administration and could assist nurses in understanding the potential for medication errors throughout the MUP.

STATE OF THE SCIENCE IN PERIOPERATIVE SAFE MEDICATION USE

The OR is a unique environment. What occurs behind the pneumatic doors of the OR takes a special skill set that is not required within many other specialties in health care. Few researchers have focused on specific problems associated with safe medication use in the OR.[23] Rather, studies have investigated other important clinical topics such as instrument and sponge counts, new technologies, fire safety, and so forth. Therefore, the literature offers very limited guidance for practitioners to improve safe medication use in the OR. Some of the earliest literature comes from researchers reporting findings collected through the Australian Incident Monitoring Study[24] supporting that system failures contributed to human errors in the unique OR setting. In fact, most of the current knowledge about medication errors in the OR stems from studies led by anesthesia, which supports why national safety experts recognize anesthesiologists as the founding discipline of patient safety.

Wanzer and Hicks,[25] using the NCC MERP taxonomy, recently conducted a review of several articles that examined medication errors in the OR (**Table 2**). This focused review provided one "look" within the unique environment of the OR as it relates to medication safety and improving clinical outcomes. The investigators indicated that the science involving perioperative safe medication use was in its early stages. They supported this claim by drawing on systematic reviews of the literature, descriptive studies, and secondary analyses because there were few randomized clinical evaluations to provide evidence. Support for their conclusion that perioperative safe medication use was in the early stages of evidence included the inconsistency of the methods used to identify errors, variations in measuring patient outcomes, and simply knowing what constituted an error.

Included in the review was a study done by Beyea and colleagues[23] that originally reported

Table 2
Studies reporting perioperative errors

Author (Year)	Setting	Design	Sample (n)
Abeysekera et al (2005)[26]	Anesthesia	Descriptive	896
Beyea et al (2003)[23]	Operating room	Descriptive	731
Currie et al (1993)[27]	Anesthesia	Descriptive	144
Fasting et al (2000)[28]	Anesthesia	Prospective design with intervention	55,426
Jenson et al (2004)[29]	Anesthesia	Review article	98
Khan et al (2005)[30]	Anesthesia	Descriptive	768
Liu et al (2003)[31]	Anesthesia	Survey	116
Orser et al (2004)[32]	Anesthesia	Secondary analysis	232
Webster et al (2004)[33]	Anesthesia	Randomized clinical evaluation	15
Wheeler et al (2005)[34]	Anesthesia	Review article	221

Data from Wanzer LJ, Hicks RW. Medication safety within the perioperative environment. Annu Rev Nurs Res 2006;24:132.

on 731 medication errors reported to MEDMARX between August 1998 and March 2002. The investigators found that 10% of the errors resulted in patient harm, including one case event in which the error was associated with a patient's death. This reported incidence of harm was nearly five times greater than the remaining cases in the MEDMARX database. Furthermore, given that the data originated from multiple institutions, it was evident that medication errors that originated in the OR were not isolated events.

MEDMARX Chartbook

The most comprehensive review to date of OR medication errors can be found in USP's 2006 MEDMARX chartbook of perioperative medication errors,[35] which examined 3773 errors in accordance with the variables of the NCC MERP taxonomy. Adding to the comprehensiveness of the data contained within the report, multiple analyses detailed the variables by age of the patient, which resulted in a more comprehensive review. The report also contained several case illustrations that further described the errors.

Based on 3773 errors in the OR, the investigators concluded that 7.2% resulted in harm, which compares unfavorably when benchmarked against the entire database in which harm was associated with 1.4% of all events. Further analyses by age of the patient suggested that pediatrics (clients younger than 17 years) had higher incidences of harm (16.7%), as did adults (11.3%) and geriatric clients (10.0%). Nearly half of the records reviewed did not include the patient age, and in this cluster, harm was present in 2.4%. The report suggested that risk of medication error

was greater in pediatrics than any other population.

Case study from the report

In one fatal case, an adult male was undergoing operative repair for a nasal fracture and facial lacerations after a bicycle accident. Following the placement of pledgets soaked with cocaine, the area was injected with what was thought to be lidocaine with epinephrine; unfortunately, he was injected with epinephrine 1:1000, which contributed to his death.

Node of the Medication Use Process

The node of the MUP was examined in 3216 records, and slightly more than half (56.3%) of the records were associated with the administering phase. As with error severity, the data supported that slightly higher percentages were associated with pediatric patients (69.4%) compared with adult (68.4%) or geriatric (68.7%) patients.

The report describes a low percentage of transcribing and dispensing errors that are reflective of the clinical practice in the OR setting. Most medications used in the OR are a result of a verbal order, or a standing order on the surgical preference card. Often it is not possible to interrupt the workflow process and write down medication orders. Likewise, this specialty setting rarely transcribes medication orders to a physicians order form as a means to process the order through the pharmacy department. Furthermore, few surgical environments have the luxury of a pharmacist dedicated to the OR. Rather, a common approach is to obtain the medications from an automated dispensing device or from open stock within the OR and then deliver the medication to the sterile field.

Case study from the report

A nurse was making a buffered solution to inject during an ophthalmic procedure. Instead of adding 1.6 mL of sodium bicarbonate to a 20-mL bottle of 2% lidocaine, 1.6 mL of sodium bicarbonate was added to 1.6-mL of 2% lidocaine and the medication was injected. The nurse discovered this error when preparing the same medication for the next case.

Type of Error

Pareto-type representations suggest that 80% of problems stem from 20% of the conditions.[36] This principle was also evident in the MEDMARX data report, given that nearly 75% of the reported errors involved only 4 of the 14 types of error selections. The most commonly reported types of errors that occurred in the OR were omission errors, wrong drug errors, prescribing errors, and wrong amount errors.

Omissions of products (meaning the medication was never given) were often associated with antimicrobial products and were typically seen in the use of intravenous piggybacks, whereby the containers were never activated or simply not infused. With regard to wrong drug administration, the leading cause of harm was related to the administration of the wrong pain medications.

Case study from the report

An elderly patient was undergoing a procedure in which a resectascope was being used. Lactated Ringer's was inadvertently hung instead of sorbitol, resulting in bleeding and increased anesthesia time.

Further subanalyses of the MEDMARX report revealed that omission errors disproportionately affected the geriatric population and that wrong amount errors negatively affected pediatric patients. The report indicated that most of the errors resulted from breakdowns in communication among health care workers following handoffs. The report also cited the failure of adequate documentation leading to medication errors.[35]

Case study from the report

A provider thought that an unlabeled syringe was an antibiotic; instead, the syringe contained a muscle relaxant. Because of the error, the pediatric patient remained intubated, which prolonged the case.

Cause of Error

The leading cause of error was performance deficit (41.8%), followed by procedure/protocol not followed (27.2%), and communication (18.1%). These findings were in line with overall trends in medication errors; however, it is important to note that other causes of errors (contraindicated/drug allergy, dispensing device involved, packaging/container design, and verbal orders) had higher percentages of occurrence in the OR environment than in the overall database of medication errors. The data further outlined the lack of proper labeling and storage and look-alike and sound-alike issues that were involved in the errors.

Case study from the report

A surgeon gave a verbal order for intravenous digoxin and misspoke the dose. The anesthesia provider did not catch that the order was a tenfold overdose and delivered the medication. An improper dose along with a verbal order contributed to the death of this infant.

Contributing Factors

Contributing factors are transient conditions (such as situational, organizational, or environmental) that alone do not lead to errors.[35] Rather, contributing factors affect the precise execution of the MUP and cause failures that result in errors. Because of the transient nature, contributing factors are difficult to anticipate, difficult to recognize, and difficult to manage.

In 40% of the medication errors reported, there was no contributing factor identified. Distractions were the highest contributing factor and accounted for 26% of the medication errors reported. This finding was not unexpected, given the dynamic nature of the work environment in the OR. Six of the identified contributing factors deal with the impact of staffing patterns on the error events. Nursing shortages have increased the use of temporary/agency staff and necessitated the need for float staff/cross coverage, resulting in the working staff being less familiar with the institution's policies and procedures. The report also identified that inexperienced staff members contributed to some of the errors.

Products Involved in Medication Errors

The MEDMARX report identified 343 different products involved in medication errors in the OR. Product classes included antimicrobials, analgesics, sedatives, and parenteral intravenous fluids. The report examined the products across populations and by errors that did or did not result in harm. The five most frequently reported products involved in harmful errors were cefazolin, heparin, fentanyl, midazolam, and morphine. It is noteworthy that of the top five products involved in errors, four were classified as "high-alert" medications as defined by the Joint Commission. Of these products, cefazolin was one of the many doses of antimicrobials involved in omission errors. With regard to central nervous system (CNS) products, errors typically involved the wrong amount being given. The most serious errors that have occurred due to the wrong product being administered include

- Excessive dose (20-fold extra) of heparin administered during a plastic surgery case, leading to loss of soft tissues
- Intra-articular epinephrine (wrong route and wrong drug), leading to cardiac arrest
- Potassium chloride administered by way of infusion pump, leading to cardiac arrest
- Vecuronium given intravenously instead of cefazolin, resulting in paralysis
- Bupivacaine given intravenously instead of infiltration, resulting in seizures
- Epinephrine (1:1000 instead of 1:10,000) injected instead of lidocaine, resulting in death
- Excessive dose (tenfold overdose) of digoxin administered to an infant, resulting in cardiac toxicity and death

Cross-Tabulation Analysis of Type of Error by Product/Class of Agent

A cross-tabulation analysis allows a deeper analysis of two variables. The MEDMARX report examined the leading types of errors and the products or classes of agents involved in the errors. The most common type of error was omission, and these errors predominantly involved antimicrobial agents. Wrong drug errors most frequently involved CNS agents. Errors in prescribing included antimicrobials, CNS agents, and nonsteroidal anti-inflammatory drugs. Errors involving the wrong amounts involved CNS agents and anticoagulants. Finally, drugs prepared incorrectly included lidocaine, heparin, and midazolam. These findings point to where quality improvement efforts can start to eliminate the burden of such errors.

Level of Care Rendered Following an Error

In 58% of the cases reported, the medication errors required no additional care. The level of care given following a medication error can range from a simple task such as increasing vital signs monitoring to the highest level of care requiring life-sustaining measures through resuscitation. It should be understood, however, that any additional care means increased resource use, regardless of whether the resources are time, supplies, or equipment. Furthermore, in today's health care industry, the outward focus is on the cost in terms of dollars. The requirement for additional tests or treatment or an increase in length of stay further increases health care costs.

INITIATIVES FOR IMPROVING PERIOPERATIVE MEDICATION SAFETY

In addition to the microsystem fixes within various clinical settings, macrosystem changes are appearing at the local, national, and health care organizational levels. These changes are becoming noticeably apparent as increasing numbers of regulatory and professional organizations are collaborating and spearheading initiatives, policies, and recommendations that are aimed at transforming the health care system into a system of safety. The Joint Commission, the IOM, the Food and Drug Administration, the Institute for Safe Medication Practices, USP, the Association of periOperative Registered Nurses (AORN), the Agency for Healthcare Research and Quality (AHRQ), and the World Health Organization along with numerous others continue to engage in systems-level patient safety initiatives in an attempt to assist

Table 3
Association of periOperative Registered Nurses Patient Safety First accomplishments related to safety

Accomplishment	Relationship to Safety
AORN standards, recommended practices and guidelines	• Recommended practice guidelines for safe medication Practices in perioperative practice settings across the life span • Guidance statement: "do not use" list of abbreviations • Creating a patient safety culture • Position statement on patient safety
AORN safety initiative	AORN Patient Safety First Event Reporting Program
AORN patient safety tool kits	• Safe Medication Administration Tool Kit • Patient Handoff Tool Kit

Table 4
Recommendations for safe medication practice

Interventions	Implementation Strategies/Rationale
Examine unit/facility policies related to medication use	Policies should Address the implementation of the read-back/repeat and verify process for verbal orders. Examine the potential of expanding the read-back process for all "standing order" medications in OR surgeon preference cards. Consider adding the element of a team review of medications to be used during the surgical procedure during the "time-out" process in relation to patient allergies and other contraindications.
Enforce a unit-based labeling policy	Ensure that all medications are labeled on and off the sterile field. Institute "leadership walk-arounds," whereby management performs spot checks to ensure the medication labeling policy is being followed.
Keep medication containers until end of surgical procedure	Ensure that staff keeps medication containers until end of case just in case there is an issue regarding medications delivered. Review all medication containers with staff during handoffs (breaks, lunch, or change of shift) as part of the medication reconciliation requirement.
Encourage pharmaceutical companies to expand involvement in product development specifically focused on the needs in the OR	To minimize errors in the labeling process, call on manufacturers to produce drug products in sterile ready-to-use packaging with duplicate sterile labels. To minimize errors seen in pediatric dose calculations, encourage the development of pediatric doses for commonly used products in the OR.
Technology purchases in the OR to improve medication safety	Obtain a buy-in from leadership who can support the need for technology purchases in the OR to improve medication safety. Examine technology that prompts documentation focused on key elements supporting the transfer of patient information and that enables the process of medication reconciliation. Have your pharmacy develop standardized dose charts that can be placed in each OR suite and readily available for staff use or purchase personal digital assistants (PDAs) for all staff, with programs to support medication calculations and formulations. Create a process to continually update the surgeon preference cards through the use of PDAs. Nursing staff could download surgeon preference cards onto PDAs, allowing "on-the-spot" changes to occur in the OR, and dock them at the end of the day to update the "system."
Patient handoff policy	Institute a patient handoff policy that improves team communication and incorporates medication reconciliation concurrently.

Review formulary for medications used in the OR	Review the facility formulary for "high-alert" medications. Standardize dosages and reduce the number of products available.
Create charts or references for staff	Outline common allergies and the associated medications that are contraindicated to those allergies. Provide a corresponding list of medication substitutions to be used when contraindications are outlined. Identify common drug–drug contraindications that are typically seen in the OR. Download these charts/references into staff PDAs for point-of-use availability of information.
Establish a "just culture"	Create a "just culture" supportive of safety. Monitor successes as improvements are made to create a culture of safety. Safety climate survey tools: www.qualityhealthcare.org www.mers-tm.net/support/marx_primer.pdf www.psnet.ahrq.gov/resource.aspx?resourceID=1438 http://www.ihi.org/IHI/Topics/PatientSafety/SafetyGeneral/Tools/ChecklistForAssessing InstitutionalResilience.htm
Implementation of Joint Commission recommendations related to medication safety	Joint Commission resources to guide safe medication use practices: Medication Management Standards National Patient Safety Goals Accreditation manual (standards) Workshops and publications
Implementation of AORN recommended practice guidelines and use of various patient safety tool kits	Practice guidelines focused on medication safety: Recommended practice guidelines for safe medication practices across the life span Do-not-use abbreviations Creating a patient safety culture Patient safety tool kits: Medication Administration Tool Kit Patient Handoff Tool Kit AORN Patient Safety First Event Reporting Program
Examine other sources for best practices in medication use	USP Web site: www.usp.org AHRQ Web site: http://www.ahrq.gov IOM Web site: http://www.iom.edu

health care organization to address medication errors. Although many of these organizations are responsible for the positive movement toward elimination of medication errors, this section focuses on the AHRQ (and their call for changing the culture of safety), the Joint Commission's initiatives, and the AORN recommended standards and practice guidelines because these three organizations have content that specifically addresses the issues of safe medication use within the perioperative environment.

Culture of Safety

Improving the outcomes of medication use requires changing the culture of the organization. The AHRQ conducted a recent patient safety culture survey that documented baseline culture from 519 hospitals. Based on 160,176 respondents, AHRQ identified that nonpunitive responses to errors was one area for significant improvement. Furthermore, the survey revealed that staff perception was that hospitals treated mistakes punitively, including filing copies of error reports in personnel files. This finding along with other data suggests that organizations are better at addressing the "individual" component of error on a regular basis (by notifying the individual, by implicating other staff members, and by providing education or training) than they are at addressing systems-level causes. This finding is not surprising, given that interventions directed at the practitioner are easier to implement. Improving the culture, however, requires removing blame from individuals and focusing attention on the root causes of the errors. In addition, the ideal culture of safety seeks out opportunities to learn from mistakes to avoid future recurrences.

The Joint Commission

The Joint Commission, formerly known as the Joint Commission for the Accreditation of Healthcare Organizations, has assisted organizations to focus directly on system changes through efforts such as the National Patient Safety Goals and the Medication Management Standards. The Joint Commission's most public parlay into quality care was the release of the National Patient Safety Goals, which began in 2002. Since then, the Joint Commission annually publishes a list of evidence- or expert-based concerns for patient safety for inclusion in the accreditation process.[37] Including the National Patient Safety Goals as part of the accrediting process elevated the importance of patients and their role in safety by directly linking the goals to the accreditation process (which is often required to receive reimbursement from the Medicare payment system). Although all patient safety goals are applicable to perioperative clinicians, goal 3 specifically calls on clinicians to label all medications and containers on and off the sterile field. This goal was developed following several serious events.

The Joint Commission's 2004 Medication Management Standards set the tone for greater emphasis on medication safety throughout an organization. The standards called for those practitioners involved in the medication management system to have readily accessible patient-specific information, such as allergy history, pertinent laboratory results, and a list of other current medications.

Another medication management standard addresses the storage requirement for medications. Organizations must also actively plan for storage of products that look alike or sound alike. An important element in this standard deals with handling of expired products. The pharmacy department must ensure removal of expired products from the clinical unit and segregate the product from other nonexpired products to ensure removal from use.

Another standard pertains to pharmacy oversight for all medication orders. Such oversight ensures appropriateness of product, dose, therapeutic indication, and a number of other safety elements. Although the 2004 standards are more prescriptive than previous standards and recognize the important role that pharmacists play in ensuring safe medication use,[38] it is invaluable for all perioperative clinicians to be familiar with the depth and breadth of the current standards.

AORN Recommended Standards and Guidelines

The IOM report To Err Is Human became the foundational stimulus for much of the activity surrounding the advancement of patient safety seen across the nation, including actions by professional organizations. The AORN, the voice for the perioperative profession, has long been a proponent for patient safety and safer medication practices. The AORN re-affirmed the profession's commitment to patient safety in 2002 after the IOM report by orchestrating several task forces charged specifically to develop initiatives, standards, position statements, and recommended practice guidelines related to staff and patient safety. One of these task forces, the AORN Presidential Commission for Patient Safety, was instrumental in creating the AORN's safety platform: "Patient Safety First," which set the framework for improving the safety of patients in surgery across the nation. This commission had a direct impact on shaping medication management practices within the perioperative setting (**Table 3**). Throughout each of these accomplishments, strategies for practice improvement were outlined in an effort to focus on system solutions to encourage organizational change. In addition, the theme of creating a culture of medication safety is woven throughout each of the documents and tools in an effort to sustain the medication error prevention strategies implemented.

Additional Recommendations for Improved Medication Safety in Perioperative Practice

In addressing recommendations to improve practice, the sky is the limit. The health care provider is limited only by his or her own creative thinking. Strategies to help enforce safe medication practices within the OR, which are founded on the information obtained from the data reports accumulated during the analysis of the MEDMARX database specifically related to the OR, are outlined in **Table 4**.

SUMMARY

Throughout this document, findings and associated recommendations for practice have been identified in an attempt to make a difference in safe medication administration within the OR. But dissemination of information is only half the battle. Lucian Leape[14] described the phenomenon of an information graveyard, whereby information becomes buried in a data graveyard if not disseminated so that others can learn and make system changes to improve safety. It takes the front-line practitioners to go the next step and to take this critical evidence and use it as supporting information to legitimize and operationalize the changes needed to successfully translate these initiatives into safety practices at institutions across the nation. The health care system needs superheros to fix the system, and the challenge is issued to the leaders within the perioperative community to become institutional champions to lead this effort for patient safety to ensure the safe delivery of medications to our patients.

REFERENCES

1. Nightengale F. Notes on nursing. Princeton (NJ): Brandon/System Press; 1970.
2. Kohn LT, Corrigan JM, Donaldson MS. To err is human: building a safer health system. Washington, DC: National Academies Press; 2000.
3. Institute of Medicine. Patient safety: achieving a new standard for care. In: Aspden P, Corrigan JM, Wolcott J, et al, editors. Washington, DC: National Academies Press; 2004.
4. Barker KN, Flynn EA, Pepper GA, et al. Medication errors observed in 36 health care facilities. Arch Intern Med 2002;162(16):1897–903.
5. Phillips J, Beam S, Brinker A, et al. Retrospective analysis of mortalities associated with medication errors. Am J Health Syst Pharm 2001;58(19):1835–41.
6. Winterstein AG, Hatton RC, Gonzalez-Rothi R, et al. Identifying clinically significant preventable adverse drug events through a hospital's database of adverse drug reaction reports. Am J Health Syst Pharm 2002;59(18):1742–9.
7. National Coordinating Council for Medication Error Reporting and Prevention. What is a medication error? 1998–2001. Available at: http://www.nccmerp.org/. Accessed April 25, 2008.
8. Rudman WJ, Brown CA, Hewitt CR, et al. The use of data mining tools in identifying medication error near misses and adverse drug events. Top Health Inf Manage 2002;23(2):94–103.
9. Association of periOperative Registered Nurses (AORN). Perioperative standards and recommended practices. Denver (CO): AORN Inc.; 2008.
10. World Health Organization. World alliance for patient safety. Forward Programme 2006–2007. 2006: Geneva.
11. Shojania KG, Duncan BW, McDonald KM, et al. Making health care safer. A critical analysis of patient safety practices. Evidence report/technology assessment number 43. Rockville (MD): Agency for Healthcare Research and Quality; 2001.
12. Wachter RM. The end of the beginning: patient safety five years after 'To err is human'. Health Aff 2004;W4:534–45.
13. Leape L. Reporting of adverse events. N Engl J Med 2002;347(20):1633–8.
14. Nyssen AS, Aunac S, Faymonville ME, et al. Reporting systems in healthcare from a case-by-case experience to a general framework: an example in anaesthesia. Eur J Anaesthesiol 2004;21(10):757–65.
15. Hicks RW, Santell JP, Cousins DD, et al. MEDMARXsm 5th anniversary data report. A chartbook of 2003 findings and trends 1999-2003. Rockville (MD): The United States Pharmacopeia Center for the Advancement of Patient Safety; 2004.
16. Shaw-Phillips MA. Voluntary reporting of medication errors. Am J Health Syst Pharm 2002;59(23):2326–40.
17. Flynn EA, Barker KN, Pepper GA, et al. Comparison of methods for detecting medication errors in 36 hospitals and skilled-nursing facilities. Am J Health Syst Pharm 2002;59(5):436–46.
18. Hicks RW. A mixed-methods analysis of pediatric medication errors from the perioperative setting. Minneapolis (MN): Capella University doctoral dissertation; 2006.

19. Forrey RA, Pedersen CA, Schneider PJ. Interrater agreement with a standard scheme for classifying medication errors. Am J Health Syst Pharm 2007; 64(2):175–81.

20. Nadzam DM. A systems approach to medication use. In: Cousins DD, editor. Medication use. A systems approach to reducing errors. Oakbrook Terrace (IL): Joint Commission on Accreditation of Healthcare Organizations; 1998. p. 5–17.

21. Hicks RW, Becker SC, Cousins DD, editors. MEDMARX Data Report. A report on the relationship of drug names and medication errors in response to the Institute of Medicine's call for action. Rockville (MD): Center for the Advancement of Patient Safety, US Pharmacopeia; 2008.

22. Legal Eagle Eye Newsletter. Medication ordered is contraindicated: court discusses nurse's legal responsibilities. 2007;15(1).

23. Beyea SC, Hicks RW, Becker SC. Medication errors in the OR—a secondary analysis of MEDMARX. AORN J 2003;77(1):122, 125–9, 132–4.

24. Runciman WB, Sellen A, Webb RK, et al. The Australian incident monitoring study. Errors, incidents and accidents in anaesthetic practice. Anaesth Intensive Care 1993;21(5):506–19.

25. Wanzer LJ, Hicks RW. Medication safety within the perioperative environment. Annu Rev Nurs Res 2006;24: 127–55.

26. Abeysekera A, Bergman IJ, Kluger MT, et al. Drug error in anaesthetic practice: a review of 896 reports from the Australian Incident Monitoring Study database. Anaesthesia 2005;60(3):220–7.

27. Currie M, Mackay P, Morgan C, et al. The Australian Incident Monitoring Study. The "wrong drug" problem in anaesthesia: an analysis of 2000 incident reports. Anaesthesia Intensive Care 1993;21(5):596–601.

28. Fasting S, Glsvold SE. Adverse drug errors in anesthesia, and the impact of coloured syringe labels. Canadian Journal of Anaesthesia 2000;47(11): 1060–7.

29. Jenson L, Merry A, Webster C, et al. Evidence-based strategies for preventing drug administration errors during anaesthesia. Anaesthesia 2004;59: 493–504.

30. Khan FA, Hoda MQ. Drug related critical incidents. Anaesthesia 2005;60:48–52.

31. Liu E, Koh K. A prospective audit of critical incidents in anaesthesia in a university teaching hospital. Annual Academy of Medicine Singapore 2003;32(6): 814–20.

32. Orser BA, Byrick R. Anesthesia-related medication error: time to take action. Canadian Journal of Anaesthesia 2004;51(8):756–60.

33. Webster C, Merry A, Gander P, et al. A prospective, randomised clinical evaluation of a new safety-oriented injectable drug administration system in comparison with conventional methods. Anaesthesia 2004;59:80–7.

34. Wheeler SJ, Wheeler DW. Medication errors in anaesthesia and critical care. Anaesthesia 2005;60: 257–73.

35. Hicks RW, Becker SC, Cousins DD. MEDMARX data report. A chartbook of medication error findings from the perioperative settings from 1998–2005. Rockville (MD): USP Center for the Advancement of Patient Safety; 2006.

36. Curry D. The pareto principle. Field Notes 2001; 10:3.

37. Joint Commission for the Accreditation of Healthcare Organizations. Introduction to the National Patient Safety Goals. 2005 (Cited on 2005 January 13). Available at: http://www.jcaho.org/accredited+organizations/patient+safety/05+npsg/index.htm.

38. Rich DS. New JCAHO medication management standards for 2004. Am J Health Syst Pharm 2004; 61(13):1349–58.

Use of MEDMARX Data for the Support and Development of Perioperative Medication Policy

Vivian M. Devine, PCNS, CNOR, RN[a],*,
Sandra C. Bibb, DNSc, RN[b]

KEYWORDS

- MEDMARX • Perioperative • Medication
- Policy • Safety • Database • Military

Perioperative evidence-based practice depends on synthesis of data from internal and external benchmarking.[1] Development of perioperative medication policy should be guided by synthesis of these data and by recommendations from perioperative professional organizations and regulatory agencies. However, limited evidence of this synthesis exists in the literature to guide policy development for safe medication practices for this critical specialty.[2] Responding to this gap in knowledge, the Association of periOperative Registered Nurses (AORN) collaborated with United States Pharmacopeia (USP) to analyze perioperative medication error reports from the MEDMARX database. This database contains a unique classification system for medication errors that supports coding of all records of medication errors according to the extent of harm, to include potential errors causing no harm. These invaluable data have the capability to guide the development of medication policy in the high-risk perioperative environment through identification of causative factors and trends. Yet, to date, there has been no descriptive summary of if, or how MEDMARX data are currently being used to support the development of perioperative medication policy. The purpose of this research study was to describe how MEDMARX data are being used to support the development and revision of population health medication policy across the perioperative continuum.

REVIEW OF LITERATURE

Population health focuses on improving health outcomes, eliminating health disparities, and reducing health care costs for a particular group of people.[3–6] Central to improving the outcome for surgical patient populations is the reduction of patient safety risk factors. The United States patient safety epidemic was documented in the Institute of Medicine's (IOM) report in 1998.[7] This landmark report indicated that 98,000 deaths occurred each year as a result of medical errors. More recently, the IOM report from November 2003, entitled "Patient Safety: Achieving A New Standard For Care," calls for a unified national health information infrastructure as a requirement to make patient safety a standard of care.[8]

Patient Safety Risk

With medical mistakes ranking sixth as the leading cause of death in American hospitals today, the

The views of the authors are their own and do not reflect the views or opinions of the Uniformed Services University of the Health Sciences, the United States Navy, or the Department of Defense.

[a] United States Navy

[b] Department of Health Systems, Risk, and Contingency Management, Uniformed Services University of the Health Sciences, Graduate School of Nursing, 4301 Jones Bridge Road, Bethesda, MD 20814, USA

* Corresponding author.

E-mail address: cdrviv@yahoo.com (V.M. Devine).

Perioperative Nursing Clinics 3 (2008) 317–325

doi:10.1016/j.cpen.2008.08.014

1556-7931/08/$ – see front matter. Published by Elsevier Inc.

urgency exists to identify probable causative factors.[9] According to recent USP data, a large portion of medical mistakes in the hospital setting are comprised of medication errors, with 235,000 errors reported in the 2003 MEDMARX annual summary report[10] and 950,000 adverse drug events reported in MEDMARX as of January 2006.[11]

In an immediate effort to decrease patient safety risk in hospitals across America, the United States Congress approved a billion dollar patient safety initiative.[12] Shortly after Congress endorsed these initiatives for all health care facilities, a plethora of literary and Web-based resources emerged. Some of these initiatives assessed and evaluated practices at both the unit and hospital level, with increased analyses of systems within health care facilities.

The MEDMARX Database

In 1998, USP created a central depository for anonymous medication error reporting through a subscription service, namely the MEDMARX database. Since then, annual reports have been published identifying common trends and causative factors among like facilities and similar groups of patients. By analyzing the trends and factors contributing to medication mistakes in various facilities, a clearer picture of the problem areas has emerged. Once identified, these causative factors could then be reduced or eliminated through evidenced-based interventions, to maximize the effectiveness of safe medication practices.

USP owns another older and less-used database for voluntary reporting of errors, named the Medication Error Reporting (MER) database. This database contains roughly one-tenth the datasets reported to MEDMARX. While it is a free, anonymous service, MER lacks the number of reports needed to generate reports of trends from its users. Although the number of medication errors should not be the sole criteria for determining a useful database, it does afford the analysis of causative factor trends.[4] Therefore, the MEDMARX database is preferred over the MER database for secondary analysis. As stated in the USP E-newsroom, "This third annual report, Summary of Information Submitted to MEDMARX in the Year 2001: A Human Factors Approach to Medication Errors, is the most comprehensive compilation of medication error data submitted by hospitals and health systems nationwide."[13]

Unsafe Perioperative Practices

The operating room and postanesthesia care unit share unsafe medication administration practices, including nonspecific policies for unit stock medications, communication of verbal orders, and written case card preference sheets. MEDMARX data have identified these specific unsafe practices in all phases of the perioperative continuum throughout the literature. Once the cause is known, systems involved in the unsafe process can be evaluated, and gaps identified, to further develop or modify existing medication policy.[2,14]

The National Patient Safety Goals (NPSG)[15] have also been created as a direct response to reported medication errors and medical mistakes, raising awareness to increase patient safety efforts. In 2005, the NPSG added reconciliation of medications across the continuum of care as their eighth specific goal.[12] This goal provides guidelines for how to achieve their recommendation, which states all patients will have a complete list of medications that they are currently taking on their chart at all times, with this information communicated throughout each phase of their care.[16] Other medication recommendations provided by this organization include improving infusion pump safety, safety of using all medications, and effectiveness of communication. This last goal is further broken down into recommending standardized abbreviations, acronyms, and symbols, as well as verifying orders through verbal or telephone orders.[12,15]

The professional organizations, AORN and American Society for PeriAnesthesia Nurses (ASPAN), have assisted perioperative advanced practice nurses (APNs) with identification of gaps within their practice environment, and have provided standardized tools to improve those patient safety, risk-prone areas. The "wrong side/site" tool kit was developed by AORN[17] in response to the Joint Commission on Accreditation of Healthcare Organizations (JCAHO) patient safety goal requirement. Additionally, the kit contained a policy template for all facilities to use, in an effort to standardize best practice policy. With the success of this interdisciplinary initiative, AORN recently developed a safe medication tool kit to increase standardization of medication practices across the perioperative continuum.

An Underused Asset

MEDMARX data are being used for performance improvement projects on the surgical population, revealing the database as a user-friendly tool.[2,18] Perioperative APNs could benefit from a comprehensive list of such studies using the MEDMARX database for a quick review of existing trends in medication errors. From this list, perioperative nurses could envision the body of evidence-based research studies available and integrate this knowledge into future medication policy and best medication practices.[19] Additionally, medication error trends that have not been explored, thus requiring further study, will be easily identified as gaps in the current body of knowledge. It is only through the exploration of these gaps that the surgical patient population can achieve a healthy, safe outcome.

Significant gaps relating to medication error causes have been identified over the past 6 years, yet there exists no collection of interventions that have been taken to correct these causative factors, as identified in medication policy documents in the literature.[2,9,10,14,20–25] Perioperative APNs are often consulted to update policy based on the latest standards, while incorporating evidence-based findings in the defense of modified policy, according to Heitkemper and Bond.[26] A list of studies in the literature using secondary analysis of the MEDMARX database to support perioperative medication policy, and assist in the identification of future research needed, would be an invaluable asset for the perioperative APN.[27,28]

The study described in this article was conducted using the methodologic approach and data collection tools piloted in a study conducted by Bibb and colleagues[6] to identify and describe clinical databases and datasets used to support development of population health programs and population health policy (**Fig. 1**). The study described in this paper focused specifically on the use of the MEDMARX data in the support and development of medication policy in the perioperative setting.

Conceptual Definition—Perioperative Medication Safety Policy

The definition of perioperative medication policy includes standards set by regulatory agencies: JCAHO, the Food and Drug Agency (FDA), and the Department of Defense Health and Human Services (DoDHHS), in conjunction with recommendations from professional organizations (AORN and ASPAN), state requirements, and facility instructions, which guide the development of evidence-based medication practices in the perioperative environment.[1,4,29]

Operational Definition—Perioperative Medication Safety Policy

Unit-based adjuncts, such as instructions, protocols, explanations, and checklists, are used to operationalize a facility's perioperative medication

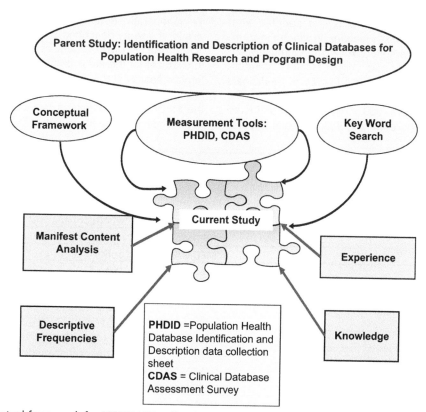

Fig. 1. Conceptual framework for MEDMARX policy document study.

policy. Specific examples of the aforementioned include laminated medication safety drug cards with preapproved calculations listed, preapproved surgeon's preference cards with desired "formulary" medications specific for the patient and case listed, and point-of-care pharmacist access.

Specific Aims

The specific aims of this study were:

- To describe the use of the MEDMARX database in the development and revision of population health medication policy across the perioperative continuum;
- To identify a list of population health medication policies that have been developed or revised, as a result of secondary data analysis of the MEDMARX database;
- To create a list of population health medication policies that could be developed and supported, using the MEDMARX database; and
- To generate a list of population health medication research topics that could be addressed for future study by perioperative advanced practice nurses.

METHODS

The research design for this study was descriptive. The methodologic approach was adopted from a study by Bibb and colleagues, in which a systematic search of the literature using the Cumulative Index to Nursing and Allied Health Literature (CINAHL) and the National Library of Medicine's search service (PubMed) bibliographic databases, covering the years 2003 and 2004, was conducted to locate completed population health studies conducted by means of secondary analysis of existing clinical or administrative data. Key words associated with theoretic definitions of clinical database, secondary analysis, military health care, federal health care, and population health programs, policy, and research were used to locate abstracts. Healthy People 2010 leading health indicators (physical activity, overweight and obesity, tobacco use, substance abuse, responsible sexual behavior, mental health, injury and violence, environmental quality, immunization, access to care) and key words "safety" and "deployment health" were also used to locate abstracts. A systematic confirmatory process and exclusion algorithm were used to determine which abstracts and corresponding articles to include in the study. A data collection template was used to guide extraction of data from each article. Descriptive statistics and manifest content analysis were used to analyze and summarize data. A total of 52 completed population health studies were included in the analysis. Twenty datasets were identified. One of the datasets identified was the MEDMARX database. Identification of the MEDMARX dataset was associated with the key words "secondary analysis" and "safety." Location and analysis of published studies associated with secondary analysis of data from the MEDMARX data set and used in the development of population health medication policy for the perioperative setting was the focus of the analysis for the study described in this article.

After the MEDMARX dataset was identified as the dataset for the focus of this study, a new systematic search of the literature was conducted to identify articles or policy documents that used the MEDMARX database in research, programs, or development of policy or policy-like documents.

Table 1
Summation of key words used for bibliographic searches

Number of Hits	Number of Abstracts Saved	Key Words
5	3	"MEDMARX" and "secondary analysis"
0	0	"MEDMARX" and "military health policy"
1	1	"MEDMARX" and "policy"
5	3	"MEDMARX" and "safety"
5	0	"MEDMARX" and "patient safety"
19	9	"MEDMARX" and "medication errors"
1	0	"MEDMARX" and "adverse drug reactions"
1	0	"MEDMARX" and "perioperative patient safety"
0	0	"MEDMARX" and "perioperative medication policy"
0	0	"MEDMARX" and "operating room policy"
0	0	"MEDMARX" and "intraoperative medication policy"
37	16	Total articles 16, minus 6 exclusions = 10 articles in study

Data Collection Process

Thirty-five key words, based on the conceptual definitions for the study described in this article, in combination with the word "MEDMARX," were used in a search algorithm to identify articles and documents (**Table 1**). A systematic confirmatory process and exclusion algorithm were used to determine which abstracts and corresponding articles to include in the study. Systematic search of the literature from January 1, 1998 through July 31, 2005 retrieved 37 articles describing the use of MEDMARX data. Nineteen of the articles were discovered through CINAHL, and 18 through the National Library of Medicine (PubMed) bibliographic databases.

The abstracts or summaries of these articles were printed to verify that they met the inclusion criteria. However, because of insufficient information in the summaries or abstracts to complete the inclusion algorithm, full articles were retrieved to determine which abstracts met inclusion criteria.

Six articles were excluded from the study because they did not meet the inclusion criteria. The remaining 10 articles were included in this study and were analyzed for content (**Box 1**).

Description of Data Analysis

A data collection template was used to guide extraction of qualitative and quantitative data from each article. Quantitative data were coded and entered into SPSS version 12.0 for statistical analysis. Descriptive statistics were used to describe and summarize quantitative data. Manifest content analysis was used to analyze qualitative data and to identify themes related to use of MEDMARX data to support policy development.

RESULTS
Presentation of Results

The first aim of this study was to describe the use of the MEDMARX database in the development and revision of population health medication policy across the perioperative continuum. None of the 10 articles included in the study contained evidence that MEDMARX data were being used to create or revise medication policy.

The second aim of this study was to identify a list of population health medication policies that have been developed or revised, as a result of secondary data analysis of the MEDMARX database. Again, none of the 10 articles included in the study contained evidence that MEDMARX data were being used to create or revise medication policy.

A summary table of all articles used in the study, with main content summarized, illustrates the gap

---

Box 1
Articles used in study

1. Beyea SC, Hicks RW, Becker SC. Medical errors in the OR–a secondary analysis of MEDMARX. AORN Journal 2003;77(1):22.
2. Beyea SC, Kobokovich LJ, Becker SC, et al. Medication errors in the LDRP: identifying common errors through MEDMARX Reporting. AWHONN Lifelines 2004;8(2):130–40. (4 ref)
3. Cousins DD. Developing a uniform reporting system for preventable adverse drug events. Clin Ther 1998;20(Suppl C):C45–58.
4. Cowley E, Williams R, Cousins D. Medication errors in children: a descriptive summary of medication error reports submitted to the United States Pharmacopeia. Current Therapeutic Research 2001;62(9):627–40. (2 ref)
5. Hicks RW, Becker SC, Krenzischeck D, et al. Medication errors in the PACU: a secondary analysis of MEDMARX findings. Journal of PeriAnesthesia Nursing 2004;19(1):18–28. (17 ref)
6. Hicks RW, Cousins DD, Williams RL. Selected medication-error data from USP's MEDMARX program for 2002. Am J Health Syst Pharm 2004;61(10):993–1000.
7. Jones KJ, Cochran G, Hicks RW, et al. Translating research into practice:voluntary reporting of medication errors in critical access hospitals. Journal of Rural Health 2004;20(4):335–43.
8. Niccolai CS, Hicks RW, Oertel L, et al. Unfractionated heparin: focus on a high-alert drug. Pharmacotherapy 2004;24(8 Pt 2):146S–55S.
9. Nosek RA Jr, Bourg MP, Pereira I. Standardizing medication error reporting using MedMARx. Legal Medicine 2002;7p, 2p. (8 ref)
10. Santell JP, Hicks RW, McMeekin J, et al. Medication errors: experience of the United States Pharmacopeia (USP) MEDMARX reporting system. J Clin Pharmacol 2003;43(7):760–7.

---

of written evidence to support policy creation and modification based on MEDMARX findings (**Table 2**).

The third aim was to create a list of population health medication policies that could be developed and supported using the MEDMARX database. To create this table, themes were extracted from all of the articles using manifest content analysis, using phrases that depicted specific medication policies throughout the articles (**Box 2**).[3,6] Generation of a list of population health medication research topics that could be addressed for future study by perioperative APNs were identified in table format (**Table 3**).

Table 2
Recommendations from the literature for medication policies that could be developed using the MEDMARX database

Literary Recommendations for Future Perioperative Medication Policy Development	No. of Supporting Articles From Box 1
1. High alert medication protocol (2nd verifier)	1, 2, 4–6, 8, 10
2. Competency evaluation of staff regarding medication policy	1–4, 7, 8, 10
3. Automated medication delivery system (decreasing reliance on floor stocked meds)	1, 2, 6, 7, 10
4. Technological System based improvements (Bar coding, built-in safety alert software, Computerized Prescriber Order Entry (CPOE), medication error reporting)	3, 6, 7, 9, 10
5. Use Point of Care Pharmacist model	1, 2, 4, 5, 7
6. Standardized acronyms, abbreviations, and medication doses	1, 2, 4, 6
7. Preprinted standard order forms with approved dosing nomograms	2, 5, 8
8. Telephone order/verbal order verification protocol with procedural steps listed	1, 8
9. Medication labeling policy of all meds (including sterile field)	1
10. Increased communication during transfer of patient (medication reconciliation)	1

DISCUSSION
Discussion of Major Findings

The major gap in the literature regarding policy change or modification supports this study's argument for an increased awareness of the use of the MEDMARX database to influence medication safety policy in the perioperative setting. This evidence-based change should be at the forefront of every APN's agenda for their individual specialty, to immediately decrease the patient safety risk through policy development. Some of the recommended policy themes are simple and can be integrated into existing policy immediately, with the more complex recommendations of system change requiring interdisciplinary resource planning.

Research topics that were identified from the literature consistent of areas within the APN's specialty that require further study. Without this

Box 2
Policies that could be developed using MEDMARX data

Standardized medication ordering system

- Computerized surgeon's preference cards with an automatic pharmacy order placed upon ordering case cart (surgical supplies)
- Built in safety alerts

Standardized medication delivery system

- Automated dispensing system to decrease floor stock for operating room and bar coding all medication

Standardized medication administration system

- Second verifier required for all pediatric and high alert medications: label all medications.
- Surgeon preference cards as dr. order for all perioperative medication

Pharmacy integration in all perioperative practices

- Preapproval of all unit formularies for floor stock
- Pharmacy involvement needed to mix medications and prepare high alert medications
- A point of care pharmacist is available

Table 3
Research topics that could be developed using MEDMARX data

Research Topic	Themes	Specifics Regarding Necessity of Research
Perioperative specialty units could benefit from research	Causative data for medication errors and near misses in specialty areas are needed	Identifies trends for harmful or near miss medication errors, and practices the following policy (ie, same day surgery, operating room holding area, and gastrointestinal/endoscopy units)
Operating Rooms could benefit from research	Operating rooms are high risk medication safety areas	Focuses on quality assurance monitors regarding perioperative policy statements, with observation and documentation data to support that the policy is being practiced
Participating MEDMARX subscribers could benefit from research	Benchmark-like institutions	Compares and contrasts medication errors in similar healthcare facilities to identify causes and examine medication policies

additional research, perioperative medication policy cannot be modified to best reflect safe medication practices for the surgical patient. Therefore, the safety of future surgical patients receiving medication rests on the APNs in the perioperative milieu and the decisions they make in modifying medication policy based on evidence-based findings.

Increased research is needed to identify specific causative factors of near misses to proactively change systems at risk to prevent medication errors from occurring. With 95% of all of the medication error reports in the MEDMARX database being "non-harm" categories, this database is the only one that should be used in the identification of preventable medication errors.[10]

Identification of Limitations

Limitations of this study included researcher subjectivity and bias, as there was only one researcher. Additionally, there was a small sample size of 10 articles.

Implications for Nursing

APNs are equipped with the skills required to analyze secondary data from nationally recognized databases for medication errors. They are also educated in recognizing areas of further research that are needed to expound the evidence-based knowledge in their nursing specialty.[26,30] The MEDMARX database contains a plethora of rich, untapped data that are waiting for someone with the expertise to recognize the immense potential in making the health care industry a safer place to administer medications. The time is now, the place is here, the database is MEDMARX, and the person is the advanced practice nurse. This is the perfect recipe for preventing future medication errors for the surgical patients of tomorrow.

Recommendations for Future Research

A list of population health medication research topics was developed that could be used by perioperative advanced practice nurses. This list can further the evidence-based knowledge of current medication policy's impact in the surgical setting. Additionally, Nosek's[9] article stated, "The Department of Defense piloted a program in December of 2000 using MEDMARX to standardize medication error reporting across the Military Health System (MHS)," and was going to report the benefits. The absence of literary evidence in this regard provides a gap in knowledge, which warrants further research to determine the effect of the MEDMARX database on medication error reporting across all military health care facilities. Further analysis of the use of the MEDMARX database in subscribing facilities through a survey would be beneficial. Additionally, further studies exploring the existence of other medication error reporting databases would add to the current knowledge base on perioperative medication safety.

In conclusion, literature does not support the modification or creation of medication safety policy based on MEDMARX database findings.

The MEDMARX database is the largest, nationally recognized medication error reporting tool available to subscribers to include the Military Health System Patient Safety Program, a Department of Defense program. These valuable data are underused in effecting change of unsafe medication policy in health care systems across the globe and should be immediately integrated into future policy decisions, with the acknowledgment as a resource. Further secondary analysis of MEDMARX data, specific to causative factors of medication errors occurring in the perioperative setting, is needed to provide the sound evidenced-based knowledge on which to develop and update safe medication policy.

REFERENCES

1. Titler PR. Nursing research: methods and critical appraisal for evidenced based practice. 6th edition. St. Loius (MO): Mosby; 2006. 439–81.
2. Beyea SC, Hicks RW, Becker SC. Medication errors in the OR—a secondary analysis of MEDMARX. AORN J 2003;77:122–34.
3. Bibb SC. Healthy People 2000 and population health improvement in the Department of Defense military health system. Mil Med 2002;167:552–5.
4. Department of Defense. Department of Defense directive: health promotion and disease/injury prevention. Available at: http://www.dtic.mil/whs/directives/corres/html2/d101010x.htm. Accessed August 22, 2005.
5. Department of Defense Tricare Management Activity. Medical management guide. Available at: http://www.mhsophsc.org?public/spd.cfm?spi=mmguide. Accessed August 22, 2005.
6. Bibb SC, Padden DL, Reilly CA, et al. Identification and description of existing datasets available for use in population health research and program design in the Department of Defense, Karen A. Rieder Nursing research poster session, San Antonio, Texas, November 2006.
7. Institute of Medicine. Institute of Medicine (IOM) report, 1998. Available at: http://www.iom.edu/?id=12735. Accessed March 28, 2006.
8. Institute of Medicine. Institute of Medicine (IOM) report, 2003. Available at: http://www.Iom.Edu/?Id=12735. Accessed March 30, 2006.
9. Nosek RA, McMeekin J, Rake GW. Standardizing medication error event reporting in the U.S. Department of Defense. Available at: http://www.ncbi.nlm.nih.gov/books/bv.fcgi?rid=aps.section.7775. Accessed October 10, 2008.
10. Hicks RW, Cousins DD, Williams RL. Selected medication-error data from USP's Medmarx program for 2002. Am J Health Syst Pharm 2004;61:993–1000.
11. United States Pharmacopeia. The MEDMARX database. Available at: http://www.usp.org. Accessed April 10, 2006.
12. National Patient Safety Foundation. National Patient Safety Foundation (NPSF). Available at: http://www.npsf.org. Accessed November 20, 2005.
13. Borden S, Gifford E. USP identifies leading medication errors in hospital emergency department. Available at: http://vocuspr.vocus.com/vocuspr30/xsl/uspharm/Profile.asp?Entity=PRAsset&. Accessed May 5, 2006.
14. Hicks RW, Becker SC, Krenzischeck D, et al. Medication errors in the PACU: a secondary analysis of Medmarx findings. J Perianesth Nurs 2004;19:18–28.
15. Joint Commission of Accreditation for Healthcare Organizations. National Patient Safety Goals. 2006;. Accessed May 5, 2006.
16. Medscape. Medication reconciliation, pharmacist involvement vital to reducing medication errors. Available at: http://www.medicalnewstoday.com/medicalnews.php?newsid=12208. Accessed December 20, 2005.
17. AORN, Medication safety tool kit. Denver (CO): AORN; 2005.
18. Hicks RW, Becker SC, Windle PE, et al. Medication errors in the PACU. J Perianesth Nurs 2007;22:413–9.
19. Hamric AB, Hanson CH. Educating advanced practice nurses for practice reality. J Prof Nurs 2004;19:262–8.
20. Beyea SC, Kobokovich LJ, Becker SC, et al. Medication errors in the LDRP: identifying common errors through Medmarx reporting. AWHONN Lifelines 2004;8:130–40.
21. Cousins DD. Developing a uniform reporting system for preventable adverse drug events. Clinical therapeutics 1998;20(Suppl C):C45–58.
22. Cowley E, Williams RL, Cousins D. Medication errors in children: a descriptive summary of medication error reports submitted to the United States Pharmacopeia. Curr Ther Res Clin Exp 2001;62:627–40.
23. Jones KJ, Cochran G, Hicks RW, et al. Translating research into practice: voluntary reporting of medication errors in critical access hospitals. J Rural Health 2004;20:335–43.
24. Niccolai CS, Hicks RW, Oertel L, et al. Unfractionated heparin: focus on a high-alert drug. Pharmacotherapy 2004;24:146S–55S.
25. Santell JP, Hicks RW, McMeekin J, et al. Medication errors: experience of the United States Pharmacopeia (USP) Medmarx reporting system. J Clin Pharmacol 2003;43:760–7.
26. Heitkemper MM, Bond EF. Clinical nurse specialists: state of the profession and challenges ahead. Available at: http://www.medscape.com/viewarticle/480355. Accessed March 6, 2006.
27. Zuzelo PR. Clinical nurse specialist practice—spheres of influence. AORN J 2003;77:361–9.
28. Nicoll LH. Policy analysis as a strategy for clinical decision making. Available at: http://www.findarticles.com/

p/articles/mi_mOFSL/is_2_70ai_55525541. Accessed March 22, 2005.

29. Association of periOperative Registered Nurses. Standards, recommended practices, and guidelines: perioperative advanced practice nurse competency statements. Denver (CO): AORN; 2006.

30. Association of periOperative Registered Nurses. Perioperative advanced practice nurse competency statements. Denver (CO): AORN; 2006.

Use of MEDMARX Data to Guide Population Health Improvement in the Perioperative Setting

Christopher R. Smith, LCDR, NC, USN, MSN, MHR, CNOR[a],*,
Sandra C. Bibb, DNSc, RN[b]

KEYWORDS

- MEDMARX • Population health improvement
- Perioperative care • Perioperative safety
- Medication safety • Patient safety

Every year, 44,000 to 98,000 persons die because of preventable medical errors.[1] Of these deaths, 7,000 are directly related to the largest subset of medical errors: medication errors. Although an actual number cannot be attributed to perioperative medical and medication errors leading to death, it is understood that errors do occur within the perioperative services.

Perioperative nurses focus on the well being and safety aspects of patient care. Their role, as the patient advocate, is to proactively assess for potential risks and then identify the systems or means to alleviate these risks. The expertise and proficiency necessary to perform at an advanced level within the perioperative arena relies on evidence-based, outcome-driven practice.[2–4] Contextually, clinical studies provided evidence-based practices aimed at improving patient care, but recent advances in information technology (in the form of health information databases) now support shifts from a focus on the individual patient to one that is focused on population health.

Population health is a proactive approach to improving the health of a population through evidence-based, outcome-driven interventions.[5] Population health data are available within a variety of health information databases and are useful for secondary analysis in support of population health research and design of interventions.

During preliminary work on a research project titled "Identification and Description of Clinical Databases," a list of potential clinical databases was identified that could be used for population health research and design of interventions. The MEDMARX database was identified as a valuable source of medication error data during this preliminary work, and was chosen as the focus of a perioperative nurse specialist-specific research project because of the relevance of MEDMARX data for population health improvement in the perioperative setting. The purpose of this perioperative-specific study was to describe the use of MEDMARX data in the support and development of population health improvement medication programs in the perioperative setting.

LITERATURE REVIEW
Population Health Improvement in the Perioperative Setting

Population health improvement focuses on decreasing morbidity and mortality through primary, secondary, and tertiary prevention.[6] Within the

The opinions expressed in this article are those of the authors and do not reflect the official policy or position of the Uniformed Services University of the Health Sciences, the United States Navy, Department of Defense, or the United States Government.

[a] National Naval Medical Center, 8901 Wisconsin Avenue, Bethesda, MD 20889, USA
[b] Department of Health Systems, Risk and Contingency Management, Uniformed Services University of the Health Sciences, Graduate School of Nursing, 4301 Jones Bridge Road, Bethesda, MD 20814, USA
* Corresponding author.
E-mail address: christopher.r.smith@med.navy.mil (C.R. Smith).

Perioperative Nursing Clinics 3 (2008) 327–332
doi:10.1016/j.cpen.2008.08.012
1556-7931/08/$ – see front matter. Published by Elsevier Inc.

perioperative arena, medication error prevention and medication safety are two very important forms of primary prevention. Although the awareness of medication errors and medication safety continues to ascend to the top of the primary health care concerns, there is little, if any, information available or research being conducted on the specific problems associated with medication errors occurring within the operating room. When information is available, it may lack the full nature, extent, and causes of these errors, which are critical pieces of information. Experts, however, agree that errors occur in the operating room and can result in serious outcomes, including death or serious injury.[7] Secondary analysis of existing medication-error data is one way to generate information useful in designing evidenced-based interventions to reduce morbidity and mortality related to medication errors throughout the perioperative continuum.

As medication errors come to the forefront of the leading health care concerns, information regarding the environment, cause, and the extent of these adverse events is paramount. Medication delivery systems can be improved by seeking a complete understanding of what constitutes a medication error and the so called "near misses."[8] A surplus of information regarding medication errors, such as which particular medications were involved in the errors, which providers were involved in medication error, and the types of errors that have occurred exists in a variety of national medical databases. The potential impact on patient safety that can be derived from this information has to be considered.

MEDMARX Database

MEDMARX is a voluntary, Internet-accessible, anonymous database that allows the reporting of medication errors by hospitals and health systems for use in tracking and trending. MEDMARX is owned and operated by United States Pharmacopeia (USP). USP is an independent, not-for-profit organization that disseminates authoritative standards and information for medicines, other health care technologies, and related practices used to maintain and improve health and promote optimal health care delivery.[9] MEDMARX supports the position that emphasizes changing the system, rather than assigning blame, will enhance patient safety. With over 850 facilities participating in the database and more than 1 million records of errors, MEDMARX is the largest database of its kind within the United States.[10] This database contains crucial information with regard to the Institute of Medicine (IOM) primary foci on the systematic prevention of medical and medication errors.[1] Hospitals that subscribe to this database are afforded access to, and can compare, medication error data with that of other health systems and hospitals. From this information, these facilities can look at error-prone environments and develop systematic improvements for implementation.

CONCEPTUAL FRAMEWORK

The conceptual framework for this study was adapted from the parent study "Identification and Description of Clinical Databases" (Principal Investigator, Dr. Sandra Bibb),[11] which proposed to identify and describe clinical databases useful in conducting population health research and designing evidence based interventions. For the purpose of this study, patient safety was defined as "the avoidance, prevention and amelioration of adverse outcomes or injuries stemming from the processes of healthcare".[12] Medication error was classified as "any preventable event that may cause or lead to inappropriate medication use or patient harm while the medication is in the control of the healthcare professional, patient, or consumer."[13] The specific aims of this study were to: (a) describe the use of MEDMARX data in the support and development of population health medication programs, conduction of population health research and the evaluation of patient safety programs associated with medication errors within the perioperative setting; (b) develop a list of population health medication programs that have been created because of information obtained from the MEDMARX database; and (c) generate a list of research topics and describe how these topics might be addressed in the future by perioperative nurses through the use of the MEDMARX database.

RESEARCH DESIGN AND METHODS
General Approach

Conduction of this study was guided by a descriptive research design. MEDMARX data-related research studies and documents (articles, programs descriptions, and so forth) were identified in two ways: through a systematic search of the literature using the Cumulative Index to Nursing and Allied Health Literature (CINAHL) and Medical Literature Analysis and Retrieval System Online (MEDLINE) bibliographic databases, and through a systematic search of the World Wide Web (WWW).

The time period for the search was set for January 1998 to November 2005. Key words relating to the concepts of population health improvement and patient safety were used in combination with the word MEDMARX. A total of

54 documents were identified initially: 24 were found in CINAHL and 30 in MEDLINE. There were 28 duplicative articles discovered between the two bibliographic databases. Of the 54 articles discovered initially, 8 articles met the search criteria.

Data Collection Tools

The Population Health Database Identification and Description (PHDID) Checklist and the Clinical Database Assessment Survey (CDAS) were developed for use in the study titled "Identification and Description of Clinical Databases" and were adapted for use in this study. The PHDID was used to guide the review of each article in an attempt to identify how the MEDMARX database is being used to support and develop population health medication programs, conduction of population health research, and the evaluation of patient safety programs associated with medication errors in the perioperative setting. The CDAS was used to accumulate the information contained on all PHDID forms.

Data Collection Process

Following approval by the Institutional Review Board, a literature search was conducted using the criteria established. The necessary steps of the search are annotated in the study framework algorithm (**Fig. 1**). After the search of the bibliographic databases was completed, a similar search of the WWW was conducted using the exact same key words to identify research studies, programs, documents, and Web sites that have

been created based on information from the MEDMARX database. Once the bibliographic and WWW searches were completed, abstracts were printed. The abstracts were separated and organized in accordance with the key search word with which they were obtained. To verify the method and results of the search, a team member from the parent study replicated the bibliographic database search and printed the abstracts that met the specifications established for the study. The results of the initial and replicated search were compared by the Primary Investigator to confirm that all abstracts met the inclusion criteria. When this step was complete, the full article published study or Web site document corresponding to each abstract was obtained. Each study was organized by date of publication, beginning with most current and regressing. All of the documents and articles that contained the exclusion criteria were reviewed and set aside. For every article or document, a separate PHDID was completed and stapled to the article or document. The quantitative data on the PHDID forms were coded and entered into a spreadsheet in preparation for statistical analysis using Statistical Package for the Social Sciences (SPSS) 12.0. Content analysis was used to extract themes relating to how MEDMARX helped support population health improvement in the perioperative continuum from each PHDID. These themes were placed into a Microsoft Word table to create a Content Analysis Summary matrix. The statistical analyses and information from each PHDID pertaining to

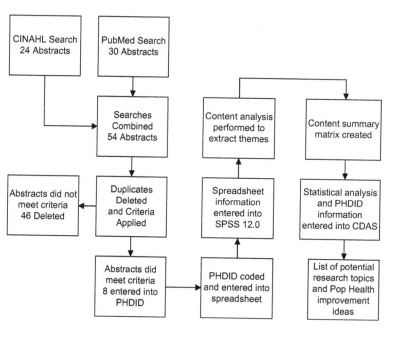

Fig. **1.** Study framework algorithm.

the characteristics of the MEDMARX database were entered on the CDAS form. Additional information needed to complete the summary form was obtained from the MEDMARX Web site. The results of the statistical analyses, content analysis, and completion of the CDAS were used to generate a list of potential research topics and perioperative population health improvement ideas for perioperative nurses.

Data Analysis

Descriptive statistics (frequency distributions) were used to describe and summarize the characteristics of articles included in the study. Content analysis was used to extract themes related to how MEDMARX data are being used to support perioperative population health improvement— only the results of content analysis are reported in this article.

RESULTS AND FINDINGS
Presentation of Results

Specific aim 1

The first specific aim is to describe the use of the MEDMARX database in the support and development of population-health medication programs, conduct population health research, and evaluate patient safety programs associated with medication errors within the perioperative setting. Data analysis related to this aim was performed using manifest content analysis. This is the process of having the researcher make inferences and categorize information based on systematic, objective, and statistical analyses during review of narrative data. Each article was read a minimum of five times to identify text, words, and concepts supporting that MEDMARX data had been used for (a) development of population health programs, (b) conduction of population health research, or (c) evaluation of patient safety programs associated with medication errors. A summary of the article titles and the authors can be found in the Appendix. Mention of population health medication programs being developed or the evaluation of patient safety programs associated with perioperative medication errors because of the information contained within MEDMARX (first and third portion of aim), was not included in the text of any of the articles. The second aspect of this aim, population health research, was strongly supported as all eight of the articles annotated some form of research, with the majority being conducted by secondary analysis.

Specific aim 2

The second specific aim was to develop a list of population health medication programs that have been created because of information obtained from the MEDMARX database. Manifest content analysis was used to identify themes related to this specific aim. After review of the literature and careful, repetitive assessment of the selected articles, no themes were identified that support the concept that MEDMARX data has been used to guide development of a population health medication programs.

Specific aim 3

The third specific aim was to generate a list of research topics and describe how these topics might be addressed in the future by perioperative nurses through the use of the MEDMARX database. Each of the articles included in the study was thoroughly examined to identify key words and recurring themes. Synthesis of the information extracted through this examination was viewed through the lens of over 16 years of experience in the perioperative arena (principal investigator of the perioperative specific study). In addition, an in-depth knowledge of the content and development of the MEDMARX database gained through conducting the systematic review for this study and careful study of the MEDMARX database by the Primary Investigator was utilized. **Table 1** is a summary of this synthesis and contains an abbreviated list of potential practice and research topics and a description of how these topics might be used or addressed for impact by future perioperative practitioners.

DISCUSSION AND IMPLICATIONS

Caring for perioperative patients is complex in nature, and today's patients have an increased attentiveness and interest in the quality of care they receive. Because of this increased awareness, many interventions have been directed at specifically addressing medication errors.[14–16] Prior to the conduction of this study, an assessment of MEDMARX data utilization for programs enhancing population health had not been conducted. Through a review of literature and the WWW, it was found that the current literature contains very limited published studies, programs, and documents that were originated based on the information contained in the MEDMARX database. These findings are congruent with the findings of other researchers.[17]

The MEDMARX database is subscriber-based and only reported to by roughly 5% of the medical facilities in the United States. This raises several

Table 1
Potential uses of the MEDMARX data to support practice or research within the perioperative continuum

Practice

Patient safety and medication safety programs	Creation of legislation because of MEDMARX information. Hospital specific programs
Unique atmosphere of the perioperative arena	Identify risk states and address in policies and procedures. Verbal communication and written documentation. Incorporate assessment for medication error into care plan. Ways to encourage error reporting.
Health care providers need additional education on medication safety	MEDMARX data use to develop and test best-practice approaches to medication safety. Safety surveys or needs assessments of patients and staff.

Research

Age-related issues of the perioperative patient	Pediatric: What does the MEDMARX data show in regards to medication errors related to children? Is there a best practice for pediatric patients to help decrease medication errors? Elderly: Are elderly patients at an increased or decreased risk for medication errors, according to MEDMARX?
MEDMARX is the largest medication error database in existence	Feasibility of a National Medication Safety Program and Repository. Is there a true need? Would it be utilized? How would it be received or viewed? Pertinence of other uses not being realized by USP/MEDMARX for patient and medication safety
Development of quality assurance indicators and improved processes	Is MEDMARX in line with recommendations of other professional organizations, such as the Joint Commission on the Accreditation of Healthcare Organizations, for example? Could it be used as to assist professional and accrediting organizations?

pertinent questions related to this article: Are the subscribing constituents of MEDMARX a true representative of all United States hospitals? Can an assessment of population health improvement be analyzed to the fullest extent? Because it is subscriber-based, is complete information of the database available for nonsubscribers? In addition, because it only represents a nominal percentage of reporting hospitals, is MEDMARX well known enough by all potential reporting entities?

Although no formal summary exists to identify studies or other documents that utilize MEDMARX, the database could become an excellent source of data for population health improvement in the perioperative setting. This database contains an inordinate amount of data available for secondary analysis or program development. The data elicited from this database will drive future perioperative practitioners in pursuit of population health-based studies focusing on patient safety and the reduction of medication errors. Therefore, further research is needed to identify future uses of the MEDMARX data and to develop concepts for prospective population health research and program development for the perioperative continuum.

ACKNOWLEDGEMENTS

The authors would especially like to acknowledge the hard work, dedication and contributions of the following persons: Lt. Col. Jorge Gomez-Diaz,

MSN, RN, Rodney W. Hicks, PhD, ARNP, and Lt. Col. Cheryl Reilly, MSN, RN.

APPENDIX: SUMMARY OF ARTICLES MEETING SEARCH CRITERIA, NEWEST TO OLDEST

Santell JP, Cousins DD. Medication errors involving wrong administration technique. Journal on Quality and Patient Safety. 2005;31:528–32.

Niccolai CS, Hicks RW, Oertel L, et al. Heparin Concensus Group Unfractionated Heparin: Focus on a high-alert drug. Pharmacotherapy 2004;24:146S–55S.

Hicks RW, Cousins DD, Williams RL. Selected medication-error data from USP's MEDMARX program for 2002. American Journal of Health-Systems Pharmacists 2004;61:993–1000.

Beyea S, Kobokovich LJ, Becker SC, et al. Medication errors in the LDRP Association of Women's Health, Obstetric and Neonatal Nurses Lifeline 2004;8:131–40.

Hicks RW, Becker S, Krenzischeck D, et al. Medication errors in the PACU: a secondary analysis of MEDMARX findings. Journal of PeriAnesthesia Nursing 2004;19:18–28.

Santell JP, Hicks RW, McMeekin J, et al. Medication errors: experience of the United States Pharmacopeia (USP) MEDMARX reporting system. Journal of Clinical Pharmocology 2004;43:760–67.

Beyea S, Hicks RW, Becker S. Medication errors in the OR-a secondary analysis of MEDMARX AORN Journal 2003; 77:122–34.

Cowley E, Williams R, Cousins DD. Medication errors in children: a descriptive summary of medication error reports submitted to the Unites States Pharmacopeia. Therapeutic Research 2001;62:627–40.

REFERENCES

1. Kohn LT, Corrigan J, Donaldson MS. To err is human: building a safer health system. Washington, DC: National Academy Press; 2000. p. xxi287.
2. DiCenso A, Guyatt G, Ciliska D. Evidence-based nursing: a guide to clinical practice. St. Louis (MO): Elsevier Mosby; 2005. p. xxxiv 600.
3. Duffy JR, Hoskins LM. The Quality-Caring Model: blending dual paradigms. ANS Adv Nurs Sci 2003; 26(1):77–88.
4. Melnyk BM, Fineout-Overholt E. Evidence-based practice in nursing and healthcare: a guide to best practice. Philadelphia: Lippincott Williams & Wilkins; 2005. p. xxvi 608.
5. Bibb SC. Population Health. In: Fitzpatrick J, Wallace M, editors. Encyclopedia of Nursing Research. 2nd edition. New York (NY): Springer Publishing Company; 2005. p. 471–2.
6. Bibb SC. Healthy People 2000 and population health improvement in the Department of Defense military health system. Mil Med 2002;167:552–5.
7. Beyea SC, Hicks RW, Becker SC. Medication errors in the OR—a secondary analysis of MEDMARX. AORN J 2003;77(1):122–34.
8. Anonymous. MEDMARX report may aid in error prevention: focus should be placed on potential errors. Healthcare Benchmarks Qual Improv 2002; 1(1):8–9.
9. Santell JP, Cousins DD. Medication errors involving wrong administration technique. Jt Comm J Qual Patient Saf 2005;31(9):528–32.
10. Hicks RW. Personal communication. 2006.
11. Bibb SC, Padden DL, Reilly CA, et al. Identification and description of clinical databases available for use in population health research and program design in the Department of Defense. Karen A. Reider Nursing research poster session. San Antonio (TX): Uniformed Services University of the Health Sciences; 2005.
12. Cooper JB, Gaba DM, Liang B. The national patient safety foundation agenda for research and development in patient safety. Available at: http://www.medscape.com/Medscape/GeneralMedicine/journal/2000/v02.no4/mgm0712.coop/mgm0712.coop-1.html.
13. Nccmerp. Definition of medication error. 1995. Available at: www.nccmerp.org. Accessed April 1, 2006.
14. Leape LL, Kabcenell AI, Gandhi TK, et al. Reducing adverse drug events: lessons from a breakthrough series collaborative. Jt Comm J Qual Improv 2000; 26(6):321–31.
15. Bates DW, Leape LL, Cullen DJ. Effect of computerized physician order entry and a team intervention on prevention of serious medication errors. JAMA 1998;280(15):1311–6.
16. Wakefield BJ, Blegen MA, Uden-Holman T. Organizational culture, continuous quality improvement, and medication administration error reporting. Am J Med Qual 2001;16(4):128–34.
17. Goeckner B, Gladu M, Bradley J, et al. Differences in perioperative medication errors with regard to organization characteristics. Aorn J 2006;83(2): 351–68.

Fire Prevention in the Perioperative Setting: Perioperative Fires Can Occur Everywhere

Claire R. Everson, RN, CNOR, CCAP

KEYWORDS

• Perioperative • Fire • Patient safety • Staff safety

A triangle is defined as a figure formed of three sides and three angles. The angles do not need to be the same degree and the sides do not need to be equal; they just all need to be present for the triangle to exist. The same can be said of perioperative or surgical fires. All three components of the fire triangle must be present for a fire to occur: heat, fuel, and oxygen. They do not need to be equal; they just need to be present. Every procedure done in a medical center, ambulatory surgery center, clinic, or physician's office has all three components present and is at risk for a fire. Throughout this article, "surgical fire" refers to a procedural fire that can occur in any health care location—inpatient or ambulatory surgery, labor and delivery, interventional radiology, endoscopy, and outpatient treatment centers, to name a few.

If you were to perform a Google search with perioperative fire safety as the search phrase, you would see 240,000 results. Stat!Ref (www.statref.com) matches to 54 documents. Depending on your search phrase, the Cumulative Index to Nursing and Allied Health Literature Web site (www.cinahl.com) can give you 30 hits. Searching for specific data for the perioperative setting from the Association of periOperative Registered Nurses (AORN; www.aorn.org) provides 35 hits. A search of the Joint Commission Web site (www.jointcommission.org) indicates 12 hits in 0.8 seconds. The Emergency Care Research Institute (ECRI Institute; www.ecri.org) matches to 21 results. In a matter of minutes, 152 sources of information are available, with an additional 240,000 if you used a generic search engine. What about finding fire safety references in the media? Again, many references were found in local and national media outlets in written and video formats.

As an educator since 1985, I have tried to present fire safety annually in creative ways, for my sake as well as that of my staff, for how boring to do fire safety education and training the same way every year. Then I was particularly struck by an ABC News *20/20* segment on March 16, 1998. This segment included interviews with victims/survivors and family members and a realistic demonstration by Mark Bruley of the ECRI Institute. At that time, this segment was available for purchase and could be used in continuing education and orientation of members of the perioperative team. Eight years later, in 2006, Mark Bruley's expertise would again be evident in the AORN Fire Safety Tool Kit. Mark Bruley, CCE, is Vice President of Accident and Forensic Investigations at ECRI Institute and has been investigating perioperative, surgical, or procedural fires for over 25 years.

Perioperative fires, although a fairly new term, are not new. In 1939, Woodbridge[1] stated,

Although statistically their importance is minute, they are of great emotional importance. The dramatic nature of the accident and of the death that may occur leads to publicity. The noise, the dramatic suddenness

Banner Desert Medical Center, 1400 South Dobson, Mesa, AZ 85202, USA
E-mail address: claire.everson@bannerhealth.com

Perioperative Nursing Clinics 3 (2008) 333–343
doi:10.1016/j.cpen.2008.08.011

and the publicity all tend to produce a wave of fear and under the emotional tension of fear it is felt that something must be done, and done quickly.

The perioperative fire is not a new problem or one specific to "modern" medicine and anesthesia. In an American Society of Anesthesiologists newsletter dated September 2000, Turner[2] briefly reviewed the history of fires and explosions, including events from as early as 1745 to the introduction and acceptance of the first nonflammable anesthetic agent, halothane. Many of these historical fires seemed caused by the fire triangle of an ignition/heat source of static electricity, inspired oxygen (or room air) mixed with a flammable anesthetic agent, and fuel. Of note was a 1930 statement by the American Medical Association Council on Physical Therapy, "A certain carelessness regarding this matter has developed."[3] Later that year, the American Medical Association Committee on Anesthesia Accidents stated, "care does not now completely forestall this hazard" and discussed the importance of "weighing the potential advantages and disadvantages of each anesthetic technique."[4]

On June 24, 2003, the Joint Commission issued a Sentinel Event Alert titled, "Preventing Surgical Fires."[5] In this alert and in other reports, there is a consensus that incidents of perioperative fires are underreported. Between the Food and Drug Administration (FDA) and the ECRI Institute, approximately 100 surgical fires with perhaps 20 serious injuries and one or two patient deaths annually are reported.[6] This figure corresponds to about two surgical fires a week. It is believed that this number is low because surgical fires are underreported; however, there is no national repository of information, and the data were teased out of reports that were sent to the FDA and the ECRI Institute; it is an estimate only. In the greater than 50 million annual surgeries, this estimated number may not seem high, unless it is a patient at your facility or the patient is someone you know. Since the advent of mandatory state reporting of surgical fires, there are hard data that the ECRI Institute uses to scale known occurrences of a single state to the United States. The current estimate is 550 to 650 surgical fires per year.

Regulations require facility accountability, and the American Association for Accreditation of Ambulatory Health Care Facilities, the Joint Commission, the Centers for Medicare & Medicaid Services, and other third-party payers are scrutinizing perioperative patient care for patient safety issues. The Joint Commission's National Patient Safety Goals, the Agency for Heathcare Research and Quality (AHRQ), and National Quality Forum "never events" contribute recommendations for patient safety, including fire safety. Many of these recommendations are evidence based and common sense, and the recommendations are similar. It is relatively easier to apply recommendations when they are consistent, no matter which reference a facility chooses to use.

At the time of the 2003 Joint Commission Sentinel Event Alert, the ECRI Institute's analysis of case reports revealed that the most common ignition sources were electrosurgical equipment (68%) and lasers (13%); the most common fire locations were the airway (34%), head or face (28%), and elsewhere on or inside the patient (38%). An oxygen-enriched atmosphere was a contributing factor in 74% of all cases.[6] When these three parts of the triangle come together in the wrong way at the wrong moment, a fire may occur (**Box 1**).

There are several types of surgery fires. The endotracheal tube in the airway may be the source of the fire. There may be a fire in the oral cavity. Fine skin hair at the surgical site may have been slicked back with petroleum jelly instead of a water-soluble jelly. The drapes may be the fire source. Equipment may also be the source of the fire. There are similarities and differences in how these may be prevented or suppressed.

The literature artificially discusses the issues as four topics. Although these topics are closely intertwined, they are divided for educational and organization of thought purposes as prevention, suppression, evacuation and communication.

PREVENTION

Part of prevention is knowledge, which is discussed later in this article.

Oxygen-Enriched Atmosphere (Anesthesia Provider)

When the patient receives anesthetic gases through a face mask or nasal cannula, there is a potential for the creation of oxygen-enriched atmosphere as the oxygen and nitrous oxide vents into the atmosphere and accumulates under the surgical drapes. This accumulation is of particular concern when surgeries are occurring in the head and neck area. The proximity of the surgical site to the oxygen-enriched atmosphere creates the potential for a spark from the electrosurgery unit (ESU), electrocautery unit (ECU), or battery-device cautery to ignite the surrounding oxygen-enriched atmosphere. In many ways ECU and ESU are used interchangeably and may have a regional distinction. However, electrocautery devices use a direct

Box 1
The fire triangle (and the affiliated surgical team member)

Heat sources (surgeon or assistant)

Electrosurgical units

Electrocautery units

Lasers

Fiberoptic light sources and cables

Sparks from high-speed surgical drills and surgical burrs

Defibrillators

Glowing embers of charred tissue[8]

Other electrical hemostatic devices

Ultrasonic hemostatic or cutting devices

Flexible endoscopes

Tourniquet cuffs

Needle electrodes versus flat-blade electrodes on an electrosurgery or electrocautery unit

Fuel sources (scrub person, circulating registered nurse, surgical technologist)

Degreasers

Flammable prepping agents including tinctures (chlorhexidine digluconate [Hibitane], thimerosal [Merthiolate]), idophor [DuraPrep])

Drapes

Towels

Gowns

Hoods

Masks

Surgical sponges

Dressings

Ointments, petrolatum (petroleum jelly)

Tincture of benzoin (74%–80% alcohol)

Aerosols (eg, Aeroplast)

Paraffin

White wax

Patient's hair (face, scalp, body)

Gastrointestinal tract gases (mostly methane)

Aerosol adhesives

Alcohol (also in suture packets)

Instrument and equipment drapes and covers

Egg-crate mattresses

Mattresses and pillows

Blankets

Adhesive tape (cloth, plastic, paper)

Ace bandages, stockinettes

Collodion (mixture of pyroxylin, ether, and alcohol)

Disposable packaging materials (paper, plastic, cardboard)

Smoke evacuator hoses

Some instrument boxes and cabinets

Oxygen sources (anesthesia provider)

Oxygen-enriched atmosphere

Oxygen delivered through a nasal cannula

Oxygen delivered through a mask

Use of flammable endotracheal tube during airway procedures with laser

Nitrous oxide

Petroleum-based jelly on eyes

Flexible endoscopes

Anesthesia components (breathing circuits, masks, airways, tracheal tubes, suction catheters, pledgets)

Coverings of fiberoptic cables and wires (eg, ESU leads, ECG leads)

Blood pressure cuffs

Stethoscope tubing

Human factors

Complacency

Distraction

Inattentiveness

Slow reaction

Improper firefighting techniques

Improper firefighting tools

Feeling rushed

current, because electrons flow in one direction through a wire. The wire provides resistance, heating up. As the hot wire is held in contact with tissue, coagulation results. ECUs are usually battery operated, such as the small disposable unit used during ophthalmic procedures to coagulate small blood vessels.[7] Seventy-four percent of reported surgical fires occur in an oxygen-enriched atmosphere.[6] When the anesthesiologist needs to increase oxygen levels because of falls in the patient's oxygen saturation, this should be communicated with the surgeon.

Heat Source (Surgeon or Assistant)

Holstering the active electrode of the ESU or ECU is a simple step that can be taken to prevent surgical fires. Traditionally a "holster" is close to the scrub person, but a surgeon may prefer the active electrode to be close at hand. Health care facilities should consider the availability of an additional holster to encourage safe practice. Providing a second holster could end the debate over using the holster versus keeping the active electrode conveniently close at hand. The risk of accidental activation by placing instrumentation or supplies (or by simply leaning) on the active electrode is also mitigated by using the holster. Mark Bruley from the ECRI Institute recommends that if the active electrode is not in immediate use (defined as 5–10 seconds), then it should be holstered or placed on the back table if it is a battery-operated device.[9]

Using standby mode is also an important step to take. The communication between the surgeon and the laser operator is one of the prevention steps to be taken. The need for laser standby mode is one of the safety reasons for staffing a separate laser operator, a person whose sole responsibility is the laser and who pays close attention to what is happening at the field and is available to communicate with the surgeon. The circulator may be assisting the anesthesia provider or opening supplies for the scrub person on the other side of the room when the laser needs to be placed on standby.

The surgeon or assistant, whoever is using the active electrode or laser delivery apparatus, should be the only person activating it. These sources should be activated when they are in contact with the tissue on which they are to be used, minimizing the potential for ignition of gases through sparks or hot currents of energy.

Communication with the members of the surgical team needs to occur when a single spark or arc is seen. The single event may not have been the only one. While the surgeon or assistant uses the active electrode or laser delivery device, respect needs to be given for the role of the scrub person in patient safety. When the scrub person attempts to holster or suggests holstering the active electrode, the scrub person should not be ridiculed or made to feel as though he or she is delaying the tempo of the procedure.

Several facilities are including fire risk assessments as part of the universal protocol. After verifying the patient's name and surgical site and marking the presence of instrumentation and implants needed, the location of the surgical site in proximity to the anesthesia gases, the safe use of heat sources, and the monitoring of supplies are discussed. This additional communication takes seconds but is a preventive strategy that should be encouraged.

Fuel Source (Registered Nurse Circulator, Scrub Nurse, Surgical Technologist)

The environment should be set up with fire prevention considerations. Knowledge of the location of fire pull alarms, fire extinguishers, and evacuation routes are part of the steps taken to prevent fires.

When planning for the intervention, the circulator and scrub person should discuss any risks that could be anticipated. Sterile saline on the field, using the holster, and the volume of music, conversation, and other ambient room noise are within their control. If the audio from the ESU generator or laser is difficult to hear over the room noise, then its volume should be raised to increase awareness of any potential inadvertent activation of the active electrode.

The staff in perioperative departments need to activate the chain of command if they believe that adequate surgical fire prevention strategies are not being taken. In reports of surgical fires, staff have stated that they were aware of potential problems but that they were ignored or ridiculed. Occasionally the assumption is made that leadership would not enforce prevention strategies, but leadership is often unaware of the problems. The staff performing the procedure cannot assume that leadership knows that prevention strategies are not being followed if they do not inform leadership. When doing leadership rounds, I am teased by some surgeons who say, "The boss is here, quick, put this in the holster." In some institutions, however, this is a serious issue.

The circulating nurse is in charge of the surgical skin preparation, even if done by a different individual. Regardless of the skin preparation agent used, the flammability hazard is decreased if the agent is allowed to dry completely. The registered nurse, as patient advocate, observes for dripping or pooling of the prepping agent and monitors appropriate drying time before draping. With the increased use of waterless gels for the surgical hand scrub, the surgeon and assistant may enter the room more quickly and stand around, perhaps impatiently, for the prepping agent to adequately dry. The circulator is empowered to confirm the dryness of the prepping agent before draping. In some institutions, the dryness of the preparation is part of a sign off or checklist and is documented.

The scrub person, as patient advocate, can delay draping until adequate dry time is allowed. This delay in draping while the prepping agent dries requires support from the leadership team. The surgical drapes may burn or melt in an oxygen-enriched atmosphere when heat is applied. Even if the drapes do not flame, melting can ignite the flammable materials below, such as towels, warming blankets, or the patient's gown.[10] When possible, the drapes should be arranged to facilitate flow of anesthetic gases to the floor. Operating rooms (ORs) require adequate ventilation and scavenger systems, but these systems are also valuable in fire prevention strategies. The use of incise drapes has many purposes, but for fire prevention strategies, it is used to decrease or prevent the oxygen-enriched atmosphere venting to the surgical site. For it to function as a prevention strategy, the seal between the incise drape and the skin needs to be monitored during the procedure.

The edges of "huck" towels used to "square off" the incision site need to be kept well away from the incision site. Surgical sponges should be moistened in saline close to the time of anticipated use so they do not dry out on the sterile back table or mayo stand. They may need to be moistened periodically while in use.

SUPPRESSION

To contain the flames, the fire triangle must be disrupted by diminishing or removing one or all of its sides (**Table 1**). When a fire occurs—flames, smoke, or fumes—the literature states that the surgical team has about 2 to 3 seconds to react and to call for help. In 30 seconds or so, a small fire can progress to a life-threatening large fire. The RACE acronym (rescue, alarm, contain, evacuate) is part of the required annual education and training. Web-based or independent learning modules are time-effective but do not assure competency. If the environment is the fire source (eg, ceiling tiles, overhead surgical lights, or smoke coming through the ventilation system), do not waste time and evacuate the patient and the team.

Rescue

In an airway fire, the anesthesia provider must shut off the anesthetic gases and disconnect the circuit if the endotracheal tube is the source of the fire. If these steps are not taken, the possibility of pulling a blow torch of flames through the trachea and oral airway is very real. The endotracheal tube should then be placed in fluid to help extinguish the fire. When the source of an airway fire is removed, immediate action must be taken to ensure that a patent airway is provided for the patient and treatment of the burned area is instituted.

When the drapes are ignited, patting the flames is ineffective—it only moves the flames in many

directions. If preparation solution dripped or pooled under the patient, the fire may be present there, too. There are different steps for different-sized drape fires (**Box 2**).

Alarm

Even when the fire is small and easily extinguished and the surgery proceeds, leadership must be notified immediately. What may have been considered a superficial drape fire may be smoldering underneath. Additional help may be needed to gather needed supplies or medications. This is not the time for the circulator to leave the room to gather them.

Policy should drive when to call the internal disaster number, when to pull the fire alarm, and when to call the fire department. It should also address who should respond to an internal department alarm and when facilities should be notified. If the facility is a free-standing ambulatory surgery center or a physician's office, the fire department should always be notified.

Contain

Keep the doors closed because the spread of a fire is always a possibility. Some containment steps were listed in **Box 2**. Do not put the endotracheal tube or removed drape in the trash too quickly because they may still be hot and a source of a secondary fire, even if the flames are extinguished. Fire extinguishers are briefly discussed later.

When discussing suppressing or working to suppress a real fire, it is important to understand that there will be by-products from the fire. Because of the materials in procedural areas, it will never simply be a fire that converts the fuel into water, carbon dioxide (CO_2), and other oxides. Incomplete combustion of materials in procedural areas may produce toxic carbon monoxide, acidic free hydrogen, and soot, ash, and debris. Plastics—hydrocarbons with other elements to create properties such as flexibility—produce the most toxic combustion products. These products include hydrogen chloride, hydrogen fluoride, cyanide, mustard gas, phenol, and aldehydes. Victims of these fires, including the surgical team, would asphyxiate before burning to death.[8]

EVACUATION

Evacuation is the last part of the acronym RACE. Horizontal evacuation of the patient and the team should be considered when the drape fire still burns on the floor, when there is a fire in the overhead lights, or in the presence of smoke and

Table 1
Suppression is adjusted by the type of fire

Endotracheal Tube Fire	Oral Cavity Fire	Surgical Site Fire	Drape Fire	Equipment Fire
Communicate with team	Communicate with team	Communicate with team	Communicate with team	Communicate with team
Shut off medical gases	Shut off medical gases	Shut off medical gases	Shut off medical gases	Shut off medical gases
Disconnect circuit	Disconnect circuit			Protect self and patient first, evacuate if needed
Extubate, removing the melting ET tube before it adheres too much to surrounding tissue	Irrigate mouth with sterile saline to put out fire	Dump sterile saline on the drapes, sponges or fuel for the fire	Pull the drapes off the patient to the ground. Roll them if possible to try to smother fire	If you can get to the electrical outlet safely, you're not in danger and no sparks from the outlet then pull the plug.
ET tube in saline or water to extinguish fire	Treat patient	Move drapes and look under them for fire	Drapes are fluid resistant so be accurate when pouring fluid on them.	If the correct, clean agent, fire extinguisher is available and you and the patient are safe, use the fire extinguisher
Control patent airway		Look under patient	Look all around and under the patient	
Treat patient		Assess patient for injury	Assess patient for injury	
		Treat patient if needed	Treat patient if needed	

Data from AORN. Fire safety tool kit: be prepared to prevent and respond. DVD education from AORN, 2006.

Box 2
Containing the flames of a surgical fire

Small flames or a small area

    Communicate to the team

    Pour normal saline slowly so the fire does not spread

    Use a towel or sponge, and with your arm between the patient's head and the fire, lay it over the flame and sweep toward the patients feet

    Lift the material used to smother the flame to vent heat

    Assess for any further flames, smoke, or fumes

    Assess the patient for any injuries and treat

Large flames or a large area

    Communicate to the team

    Remove the drape to the ground, rolling it on itself to smother the fire

    Do not move the drape into what may need to be your evacuation route from the room

    Assess the surgical field for a secondary fire of the underlying drapes or towels

    Assess the patient for injury and treat

    Circulator assures the flames are extinguished, which may include the use of a fire extinguisher

Data from AORN. Fire safety tool kit: be prepared to prevent and respond. DVD education from AORN, 2006.

---

fumes. Communication needs to occur so that the plan is known to all, including the rest of the department. The evacuation may be as simple as moving to a different OR or to a separate fire compartment, or be as complex as a department evacuation. When the decision to evacuate is made, communication will also contain the risk of the fire spreading externally from the room (**Table 2**).

Understanding the evacuation plan may be more complex than was anticipated during the annual review. It is not just knowing the "route" but knowing what to do if the route is blocked—where to take the patient and how to move the patient if he or she is on a fracture table or during a robotic procedure. The complexities of the environment are individual to each department, so they need to be discussed. The 2006 AORN Fire Safety Tool Kit includes tools that can be used when planning facility evacuation plans in detail.

It must be faced that there may be an occurrence of fire in which the fire involving the patient is too huge or the smoke is too dense or the fumes are too overpowering, and all the staff can do is save themselves. If this happens, those staff members will need support as they face and work through this tragedy. It is senseless to add to the victim count in such occurrences.

COMMUNICATION

Communication of the fire plan needs to be constant and is important in the prevention and suppression of fires and in the safe evacuation of the entire team. Because surgical fires are rare occurrences, simulation training and annual drills with debriefing sessions are critical.

The time to communicate during a fire is limited and valuable. Although it is human to ask, "What do we do?" in this rare event, the communication time needs to be better spent. Rather than asking the question, it is suggested that each team member communicates what they are actively doing.

Communication used as a preventive step is so much easier than trying to communicate during a fire. The perioperative team should communicate verbal confirmation that the preparation is dry before draping and of heat source standby, the use of holsters, when the anesthesia provider adjusts oxygen flow, when the surgeon is going to use a heat source, and what the risk of a surgical fire may be.

Another critical, although uncomfortable, communication needs to be addressed. As patient and family advocates, we need to be aware of the impact that a surgical fire will have on the patient and his or her family and friends. Realizing that they have a different perspective should direct our discussions with them. The surgeon may have the initial contact, but there needs to be a plan for a representative from the facility to communicate with them. The options include administration and risk management personnel; however, perioperative leadership may be better able to answer technical questions. What families share by way of interviews and blogs is the frustration they experience when no one seems to know what is happening, or the family feels they are being ignored because the facility fears legal action. Families could benefit from knowing that their health care team is also frustrated, because surgical fire occurrences are rare and there may not be a pre-existing care plan beyond RACE. This frustration led one family to develop the Web site www.surgicalfire.org in fulfillment of their mother's wishes.

Table 2
Different personnel have complementary evacuation steps that need to be taken

Surgeon	Scrub Person	Anesthesia Provider	Circulator
Stabilize surgical site	Protect the surgical site	Shut off anesthesia machine and gases	Communicate the need to evacuate that room to the department
Prepare site for transport, pack with sponges, cover with towels	Gather necessary instruments and sponges	Breakdown monitors, leads, prepare airway and IVs for move	Assist with preparing the patient to move
Final directions to circulator	Assist in moving the OR table	Stabilize patient, gather needed medications	Help move the OR table
Assist in moving the OR table		Coordinate move of the OR table after unlocking it	

Data from OR surgical fire training: how to prevent and respond to surgical fires. DVD education from hcPro, 2005.

ORIENTATION AND ONGOING, ANNUAL EDUCATION AND COMPETENCY ASSESSMENT

Issues to be addressed include many topics that do not come readily to mind in the 2- to 3-second reaction time allowed in the event of a perioperative fire. Education and training of staff is mandated by every regulatory agency. Not only do registered nurses and surgical technologists need this education and training but the surgeons, anesthesia providers, anesthesia technicians and technologists, orderlies, nursing assistants, and unit clerks also should participate. In addition, vendors (health care industry representatives), radiology technologists, and students should be included in annual education and drills. Points to include are fire risk, prevention, risk reduction, suppression strategies, and the development of policies, procedures, and evacuation plans.

The content of orientation and continuing education is strongly suggested in many regulatory manuals. The 2005 AORN guidance statement, "Fire Prevention in the Operating Room," is an available, helpful tool.[11]

When a "fire map" is used as an orientation tool, the location of the extinguishers, exits, pull alarms, evacuation devices, and fire doors should be located and placed on the map by the new employee.

CONDUCTING FIRE DRILLS

Evidence supports simulation training for increased retention of information and performance response afterward. A fire drill should occur annually, followed by a debriefing. Drills for evacuating the OR in the event of a major fire and surgical team drills for fighting fires involving the patient are rare but should not be.

Although meeting fire safety training requirements in an effective, realistic, and capable manner is difficult because of the many demands on the OR staff, having a preplanned method of fighting a surgical fire so that every team member knows what to do is critically important. Simulation should include the inevitable problems that arise during emergencies, such as exits that are blocked, equipment that is not working, rooms that are crowded with people and equipment, and surgical tables that are difficult to move. The simulation and training should include the following:

Keeping minor fires from getting out of control
Managing fires that do get out of control
Location and proper use of firefighting tools; medical gas valves; heating, ventilation, and air-conditioning controls; and electrical supply switches
Fire alarm and communication system

All fires start small. Surgical teams should be trained in and practice drills for quickly stopping small fires that involve drapes, gauze, ointments, and liquids. But fires move quickly, and slow reactions or confusion can allow a small fire to become a large, more dangerous one. Large fires, especially, require special drills devoted to developing the team effort needed to deal with sizable volumes of flame and smoke and with burning drapes and plastic in the small space of an OR.[8]

Fire extinguishers are critical to managing fires, and staff should be trained in their proper use. Drills should identify the location of medical gas, ventilation, and electrical systems and controls and when, where, and how to shut off these systems. The fire-containment design and construction of most hospitals helps to ensure that the staff has enough time to evacuate other patients and staff. The use of the hospital's alarm system and system for contacting the local fire department should also be defined.

The debriefing to review errors made in the drills is vital. In one of the author's earlier fire drill experiences, the operator never notified the fire department, not knowing that the drill had been coordinated with the fire department who was waiting for the call across the street in a parking lot. In subsequent drills, staff were included who were "injured" but ignored as other staff evacuated the "patient." In a later drill, the e-cylinder delivery person brought in his cart of oxygen tanks. As an observer, I informed him that he had just died in an explosion and that the explosion had spread fire to the other levels. Although he was aware of the alarm chimes, he ignored them because it was October, Fire Safety Month, and he "knew" it was just a drill.

The team influences the fire triangle; therefore, it is wise to identify a physician champion and a facilitator because the team needs to write the policy and practice guidelines.

Who orders and who uses the gas shut-off valves for the department or the individual OR? Although evacuation is horizontal, where should the patient be taken horizontally? Developing a policy or practice guideline after your first drill may be beneficial because the multidisciplinary team may realize the real need for this collaboration.

USING FIRE EXTINGUISHERS

Fire extinguishers are classified according to National Fire Protection Association standards as Class A (for wood, paper, cloth, and most plastics), Class B (for flammable liquids or grease), or Class C (for energized electrical equipment).

The various types of fire extinguishers available to fight each class of fire are described in the following paragraphs. Knowing how these devices work and when to use them will minimize the disaster of an OR or surgical patient fire.

Carbon Dioxide

A 5-lb CO_2 fire extinguisher is the best choice for putting out fires typically encountered in ORs, where the patient is the primary concern. Despite their Class BC rating, CO_2 extinguishers can be used to extinguish small masses of cloth, plastic, or paper (Class A) involved in patient fires, and

any flammable liquid (Class B) or electrically energized (Class C) fires that could occur in the OR. Equally important, these extinguishers do not leave residue and will not harm the patient, staff, or equipment. A 5-lb capacity CO_2 extinguisher weighs approximately 7 to 9 kg (15–20 lb), fits in a space approximately $23 \times 23 \times 36$ cm ($9 \times 9 \times 14$ in), and is easily handled by most people. For easy access, the extinguisher should be mounted inside the OR near the entrance.[8]

Dry Powder

Class ABC-rated fire extinguishers are not appropriate for use in the OR. These models disperse a cloud of fine, dry powder (usually ammonium phosphate) that extinguishes the fire. This cloud contaminates all surfaces in the OR, including the patient and any surgical wounds. In addition, the powder is a respiratory irritant, which could affect the staff's ability to aid the patient, is hard to remove from wounds, and requires that all contaminated equipment be thoroughly cleaned. Although dry powder extinguishers should be available in the OR suite (outside individual ORs), they should be used in the OR only as a last resort.[8]

Halon

Halon extinguishers consist of hydrogenated halocarbons and are preferred for laser unit fires. They were of environmental concern at one time but an environmental friendly halon fire extinguisher that does not negatively affect the ozone layer is now available. These units have a unique fire extinguishing action (disrupting the flaming process) and a low weight, making them easy to use.[12]

Water

Pressurized-water (PW) fire extinguishers are available, but they are heavy and chiefly effective against Class A fires. Using a PW extinguisher is more difficult to use than a halon or CO_2 device. To extinguish burning water-repellent drapes with a PW fire extinguisher, users must place a finger partially over the end of the nozzle to produce a fine spray. Water in a stream or tossed from a pan can fan the flames and increase a drape fire. Water from corridor-located fire hoses typically spray 50 gallons of water a minute and can be effective as a last resort when immediate rescue or evacuation is needed.

Water as a fire-extinguishing agent can be used over a wide range of fires; however, a fire involving energized electrical equipment, although rare in the OR, should be extinguished not with water but with an extinguisher rated for Class C fires.[8]

Proper Use

Local fire departments may provide the staff with hands-on practice in extinguishing real fires using the equipment available in the OR. This training is valuable to free-standing locations that may not have a facility services department who would be the initial fire response team and would teach staff the use of fire extinguishers. A return demonstration helps build the familiarity and confidence needed to use these devices in a frightening and hectic situation. Fire extinguishers should be small enough to be easily carried and handled by the most likely users, and they should be located in plain view in positions of easy access—near escape routes but away from fire-hazardous areas. Most fire extinguishers are operated according to the following procedure, whose steps are abbreviated by the acronym "PASS."

> Pull the activation pin.
> Aim the nozzle at the base of the fire.
> Squeeze the handle to release the extinguishing agent.
> Sweep the stream over the base of the fire.

Summary

Surgical, perioperative, and interventional procedures, no matter where they are performed and no matter what we call them, are never a no-risk situation, and the potential for a fire should always be recognized. Free-standing ambulatory surgery centers, endoscopy centers, imaging centers, and physician's offices have gaps in emergency services and response teams. These areas need well-understood plans, intense orientation, and ongoing education because there is no one else to rely on until the fire department arrives.

ECRI INSTITUTE RECOMMENDATIONS

> Staff should question the need for 100% oxygen for open delivery during facial surgery and, as a general policy, use air or fraction of inspired oxygen at <30% for open delivery (consistent with patient needs).
> Do not drape the patient until all flammable preparations have fully dried.
> During oropharyngeal surgery, soak gauze or sponges used with uncuffed tracheal tubes to minimize leakage of oxygen into the oropharynx and keep them wet; moisten sponges, gauze, and pledgets (and their strings) so that they will resist igniting.
> When performing electrosurgery, electrocautery, or laser surgery, place electrosurgical electrodes in a holster or other location off

the patient when not in active use; place lasers in standby mode when not in active use.

In addition, the ECRI Institute recommends that staff should participate in special drills and training in the use of firefighting equipment; the proper methods for rescue and escape; the identification and location of medical gas, ventilation, and electrical systems and controls and when, where, and how to shut off these systems; and the hospital's alarm system and the system for contacting the local fire department.

JOINT COMMISSION RECOMMENDATIONS

The Joint Commission recommends that health care organizations help prevent surgical fires by

> Informing staff members, including surgeons and anesthesiologists, about the importance of controlling heat sources by following laser and ESU safety practices
> Managing fuels by allowing sufficient time for patient preparation
> Establishing guidelines for minimizing oxygen concentration under the drapes
> Developing, implementing, and testing procedures to ensure appropriate response by all members of the surgical team to fires in the OR
> Raising awareness and ultimately preventing the occurrence of fires in the future by reporting any instances of surgical fires; reports can be made to the Joint Commission, the ECRI Institute, the FDA, and state agencies, among other organizations

REPORTING SURGICAL FIRES—THE LEGAL REQUIREMENTS

Many states and some professional organizations have regulations or standards requiring hospitals to report fires to their local fire department. From a risk management point of view, the safest course is to notify the fire department and keep records of any fire in your hospital. Clinical department heads should notify the safety officer, the hospital risk manager, and the hospital administrator in the event of a fire.

In addition, the event should be analyzed to determine whether it must be reported to FDA under the Safe Medical Devices Act. For example, in the case of a laser-related injury to a patient, a report would be required and the issue should be discussed with the hospital's risk manager. Many facilities bring in external experts (eg, the ECRI Institute or Russell Phillips & Associates) to help with the systematic review. The risk manager will have current information about who needs to be or who should be notified in case of a surgical fire. In reporting and reviewing, the event can be drilled down to its basic causes and the entire health care community can learn from another's experience.

FURTHER READINGS

2008 National Patient Safety Goals. The Joint Commission. Available at: http://www.jointcommission. org/GeneralPublic/NPSG/08_npsgs.htm.

Accreditation Handbook for Ambulatory Health Care. Accreditation Association for Ambulatory Health Care, Inc. 2008. Available at: http://www.aaahc. org.

AORN tool kit promotes perioperative fire safety. AORN Connections. 2006;4(1):1, 9.

Cantrell S. Fanning the flames of surgical fire prevention. Healthcare Purchasing News, May 2008. Available at: http://www.hpnonline.com/inside/ 2008-05/0805-OR-Fire.html.

Department of Health and Human Service. Federal Register. Vol. 68, No. 7. January 10, 2003. Rules and Regulations.

Department of Health and Human Service. Federal Register. Vol. 70, No. 57. March 25, 2005. Proposed Rules.

Electrosurgical units and the risk of surgical fires. Pennsylvania Patient Safety Reporting System Patient Safety Advisory 2004;1(3):9–10.

Health and Safety Issues in Operating Rooms. Building Knowledge. September 18, 2007.

Leamy, E. Could you catch fire during surgery? Fires can break out in the operating room. ABC News July 20, 2006. Available at: http://abcnews.go. com/GMA/Consumer/story?id=2215961&page=1.

Practice Advisory for the Prevention and Management of Operating Room Fires. A report by the American Society of Anesthesiologists Task Force on Operating Room Fires. May 2008, 108:5.

Risk of fire from alcohol-based solutions. Pennsylvania Patient Safety Reporting System Patient Safety Advisory 2005;2(2):13–4.

Three "Never Complications of Surgery" are hardly that. Pennsylvania Patient Safety Reporting System Patient Safety Advisory. 2007;4(3):82.

REFERENCES

1. Woodbridge PD. Incidence of anesthetic explosions. JAMA 1939;113:2308–10.
2. Turner K. Fires and explosions. ASA Newsl 2000;64(9). Available at: http://www.asahq.org/Newsletters/2000/ 09_00/fires0900.htm.
3. William HB. The explosion hazard in anesthesia. JAMA 1930;94:918–20.
4. Henderson Y. The hazard of explosion of anesthetics. JAMA 1930;94:1491–8.
5. The Joint Commission. Sentinel Event Alert. Preventing surgical fires 2003;29 Available at: http://www. jointcommission.org/SentinelEvents/SentinelEvent Alert/sea_29.htm.
6. ECRI. A clinician's guide to surgical fires: how they occur, how to prevent them, how to put them out [guidance article]. Health Devices 2003;32(1):5–24.
7. Alexander's care of the patient in surgery. 13th edition.
8. ECRI. The patient is on fire! A surgical fires primer. Medical safety devices report. Guidance 1992; 21(1):19–34.
9. AORN. Fire safety tool kit: be prepared to prevent and respond. DVD education from AORN 2006;. Available at: http://www.aorn.org/PracticeResources/ToolKits/ FireSafetyToolKit.
10. OR surgical fire training: how to prevent and respond to surgical fires. DVD education from hcPro, 2005. Available at: http://www.aorn.org/ PracticeResources/ToolKits/FireSafetyToolKit.
11. AORN. Guidance statement: fire prevention in the operating room. AORN standards and recommended practices. Denver: AORN Publications; 2008. p. 171–9.
12. Ball KA. Laser biophysics, systems and safety. In: Lasers: the perioperative challenge. 3rd edition. St. Louis, MO: Mosby; 2004. p. 76–84.

Bloodless Surgery and Patient Safety Issues

Jarrell Fox*, Sandy Brown, RN, Rebecca Vigil, RN

KEYWORDS

- Transfusion • Bloodless • Surgery
- Transfusion-free • Safety • Ethics
- Alternatives • Conservation • Anemia • Bleeding

"Bloodless" surgery? "NO BLOOD!" These requests and demands most certainly have an impact on patient safety and quality of care in the surgical setting. Have you wondered why there is an increasing international interest in nonblood medical and surgical management of patients? The answer may be surprising. Can those in the health care profession safely and compassionately accommodate patient requests to avoid blood transfusion?

The perception within the medical community is that when patients refuse blood, those patients actually are refusing reasonable medical care. This leaves patients and the medical personnel feeling frustrated. The medical professionals (physicians and nurses) believe they are facing an unnecessary barrier to traditional medical care, whereas patients feel frustrated at a perceived indifference to their personal beliefs.[1]

It is the authors' experience that the increased demand for nonblood medical care is not limited to those who have a religious objection to its use. The principal reasons include a deeply held religious belief, personal concerns about the perceived risks involved, an increased awareness of available alternative strategies, and inadequate availability of safe blood products.

Blood products, as therapeutic agents, have been used routinely for decades but lack clinical trials and regulatory review by the Food and Drug Administration (FDA) required for other products used in medicine.[2] Blood is classified as a specialized form of connective tissue. Therefore, a blood transfusion should be viewed as an organ transplant because it is living tissue. It often is viewed and prescribed, however, more like a pharmaceutical agent by medical professionals. The most common published risk from blood transfusion, blood delivery error, supports the notion that blood is handled as a pharmaceutical agent.

Over the past few decades, the risk for associated complications with blood transfusion has raised safety concerns in the public and medical and regulatory arenas. At the same time, data from clinical trials and medical practice have been collected looking at the outcomes of patients who refused blood versus those who received blood transfusion. This has brought to light positive outcomes achieved by using alternative modalities in the perioperative setting to reduce or avoid blood transfusions. These include improved patient outcomes,[3,4] shorter lengths of hospitalization,[5] reduced infection rates,[6,7] and significant cost savings.[8]

These data also reveal a variance of transfusion practice between individual physicians and hospitals and demonstrate the need to standardize blood use protocols and procedures. Time and again in research and clinical experience, there is found justification for revisiting a professional point of view on the use of blood transfusions.

The American Association of Blood Banks' *Circular of Information for the Use of Human Blood and Blood Components* states, "red cell-containing components should not be used to treat anemia that can be corrected with specific medications."[9] Dr. Paul Hébert, critical care specialist at Ottawa General Hospital, Canada, agreed with the conclusion drawn in the publication, after completing a landmark study on the effectiveness of blood transfusion practices on critically ill patients suffering from anemia. The study compared patients

Transfusion-Free Medicine and Surgery Program, Franciscan Health System, St. Joseph Medical Center, 1717 South J Street, Tacoma, WA 98405, USA
* Corresponding author.
E-mail address: jarrellfox@fhshealth.org (J. Fox).

Perioperative Nursing Clinics 3 (2008) 345–354
doi:10.1016/j.cpen.2008.08.005

treated with liberal and those treated with more restrictive transfusion policies. He summarizes, "We've been transfusing blood for 50 years and no one's ever bothered to find out how much to give. Now we know it's safe to transfuse less."[10]

It is increasingly apparent that, at the very least, less risky options should be considered before resorting to the use of blood, but the question is, are they? Ask yourself, what is the medical facility's standard of care for treating anemia? What is my reaction when I see a patient's laboratory report of a hemoglobin (Hgb) level of 8 or 9? How do I react when a patient makes a request for alternatives to a professional recommendation of transfusion? An appropriate reaction to this request may require a paradigm shift within a health care institution and among individual health care professionals. Education is a key factor in accomplishing this shift. This article hopes to provide insight into the emerging and fascinating field of transfusion-free medicine and surgery.

Major medical centers around the world have successfully implemented nonblood strategies and techniques with dramatic and even impressive results. A successful approach incorporates the collective efforts of a multifaceted team, including skilled physicians and surgeons, capable and compassionate nurses, supportive hospital administration, and appropriately equipped medical facilities.

MEDICAL ETHICS

Medical professionals are committed to applying their knowledge, skills, and experience in fighting disease and death. What health care providers believe is in the best interest of patients may not be what patients believe is best. Patients may have more holistic concerns that include their emotional, psychologic, social, spiritual, and physical well-being. Whether or not a medical professional agrees with patients' decisions to refuse blood, one has the responsibility to support patients in their constitutional right to refuse medical care just as if it were an aspirin or chemotherapy agent that they were refusing.[11] According to Appelbaum and Roth, 19% of patients at teaching hospitals refused at least one treatment or procedure, even though 15% of such refusals "were potentially life endangering."[12]

As John Stuart Mill aptly wrote, "No society in which these liberties are not, on the whole, respected, is free, whatever may be its form of government... Each is the proper guardian of his own health, whether bodily, or mental and spiritual. Mankind are greater gainers by suffering each other to live as seems good to themselves, than by compelling each to live as seems good to the rest."[13]

Case Study 1

An otherwise healthy 57-year-old female patient presents to an emergency room, having had right-sided abdominal pain and flu-like symptoms for 5 days. Diagnostic laboratory results indicate Hgb of 10.5, hematocrit (Hct) of 31%, and mildly elevated white blood cell count. CT scan confirms suspected appendicitis. The patient is prepped for emergent appendectomy. The on-call general surgeon, on seeing the patient and learning that she is one of Jehovah's Witnesses, refuses to do the surgery because of her religious objection to the use of blood transfusions. The physician neither contacts another surgeon to transfer patient care nor writes an order for pain medication. The hospital's house supervisor is not able to find an alternate surgeon on staff to accept the case. Their affiliated hospitals are contacted and their on-call surgeons also decline the case.

Was this case handled ethically? Did the physician have a reasonable concern? Was there a way to accommodate the patient's request without violating the surgeon's personal ethics?

Ultimately the patient was medicated by an anesthesiologist and a nurse arranged transfer by ambulance to a local facility with a transfusion-free medicine program. This facility's on-call general surgeon consulted with the patient and her family and proceeded to surgery promptly. During the laparoscopic surgery it was discovered that the appendix had ruptured. The patient subsequently recovered from surgery and was discharged on postoperative day 2.

Thankfully, the views of the first surgeon are not shared by all surgeons. Remmers and Speer, when discussing medical care of the Jehovah's Witness patient population, highlighted that surgical and medical procedures once considered too risky for Witness patients "are now performed routinely with few complications." The referenced literature includes reports of successful complex cardiac surgeries and pancreas, liver, and bone marrow transplantation. They note that the willingness of physicians to accommodate Witness patients' request for "bloodless medicine" has led to great medical progress in transfusion medicine and blood conservation.[1]

First do no Harm

It is the goal of ethically responsible health care professionals to help and to heal people, not to inflict harm. Therefore, we must always ask ourselves, does the benefit outweigh the risk? Does the informed patient agree?

ASSOCIATED RISKS FROM TRANSFUSION

Rachel Womak[4] recently reported in *New Scientist*, "Over the past decade a number of studies have found that, far from saving lives, blood transfusions can actually harm many patients. The problem is not the much-publicized risk for blood-borne infectious agents, such as HIV and hepatitis, but the blood itself." Study after study has shown that transfusions, particularly those containing red blood cells, are linked to higher death rates in patients who have had a heart attack, undergone heart surgery,[14] or who are in critical care. The exact nature of the link is uncertain, but it seems likely that chemical changes in ageing blood, their impact on the immune system, and the blood's ability to deliver oxygen are key.

Most experts now agree that the risk posed by the transfused blood itself is far greater than that of a blood-borne infection. "Probably 40 to 60 per cent of blood transfusions are not good for the patients," says Bruce Spiess, a cardiac anaesthesiologist at Virginia Commonwealth University in Richmond.[4] "There is virtually no high-quality study in surgery, or intensive or acute care—outside of when you are bleeding to death—that shows that blood transfusion is beneficial, and many that show it is bad for you," says Gavin Murphy, a cardiac surgeon at the Bristol Heart Institute.[4]

Disease Transmission

Although blood transfusion is considered "safer than it has ever been,"[15] making a safer end product has meant increased cost and reduced supply of "acceptable" blood products. These "safer" transfusions still carry an inherent, although minimal, risk for transfusion-transmitted infections and an evermore apparent risk for emerging pathogens.

Immunomodulation

Neil Blumberg, MD, an authority on transfusion medicine and hematology estimated that 10,000 to 50,000 persons in the United States die each year as a result of transfusion-related immunomodulation.[16] Clinical trials consistently demonstrate an association between the number of transfusions and an increased number of nosocomial infections and multiple organ failure.[16] The evidence to date gives us proof beyond a reasonable doubt that there is reason to proceed with caution.[17]

Human Error

A greater and less appreciated risk than acquiring disease is human error, which reportedly occurs in closer to 1:1000 transfusions. This error can be fatal if it results in the hemolytic reaction associated with ABO incompatibility, which reportedly occurs in 1:100,000 transfusions.[18]

Limitations of the Screening Tests

Screening is only as reliable as donors are in answering a screening questionnaire honestly. In an effort to make the blood supply safe, nucleic acid testing has helped in reducing the window period of some of the markers for HIV/AIDS and hepatitis C virus in which these cannot be detected. The risk, however, is not zero. One need only review the FDA blood product recall lists to see that blood donated by high-risk individuals still makes it into the blood supply.

PROFESSIONAL CONSIDERATIONS

Given the ethical considerations and associated risks from transfusion, how can health care professionals safely deliver care to this patient population? For bloodless or transfusion-free care to be accomplished safely and successfull, three phases of patient care must be integrated vigilantly. These three phases are (1) preoperative evaluation and preparation, (2) intraoperative strategies and techniques, and (3) postoperative monitoring and care.

It has been said that one of the most important roles of a nurse is to listen carefully, be observant, and notice things. This could not be more true than in the perioperative setting. Some things that otherwise might tend to go unnoticed could be indicators that patients are in danger. In each of the three phases, it is imperative to continually assess the patient condition and alert the team to possibly significant changes. Patient assessment and management of anemia throughout these phases is discussed, and associated recommendations are offered for consideration in each phase. Relying on nurses' knowledge, experience, and instinct is vital a factor in caring for these patients safely and integral in avoiding unnecessary complications.

PREOPERATIVE CONSIDERATIONS
Medications/Supplements/Herbs

Is a patient on anticoagulants (eg, warfarin) or antiplatelet drugs (eg, clopidogrel or ticlopidine)? Many patients often do not mention taking Alka-Seltzer, as they do not realize that it contains aspirin.

Is a patient currently taking any of the following supplements or herbs that may contribute to increased bleeding times: ginkgo biloba,[19] garlic, cayenne, ginger, ginseng, and quinine?[20]

Physical and Medical History

A thorough history and physical should be performed well in advance of the surgery. Do patients have any personal or family history of bleeding disorders or risk factors that might increase bleeding tendency? Contraindications to an elective surgery might include acute infection, anemia, or clotting disorders. Just as an elective surgery likely would be cancelled for an acute infectious process so too consideration should be given to rescheduling when patients have an uncontrolled clotting disorder or an anemia. Ideally these would be identified and treated well before the day of surgery. Nevertheless, if first noted on the day of surgery, a nurse has a responsibility, as patient advocate, to notify the surgeon or anesthesiologist of the concern and possibly recommend rescheduling. The physician then would weigh the expected blood loss in light of the patient's hematologic status (Hgb, Hct, platelet count, iron studies) and determine the patient's ability to accommodate the blood loss safely. If it is determined that surgery should be postponed, what can be implemented to optimize the patient's condition for a future surgery?

Active Bleeding?

If patients have gross active bleeding, surgery may be warranted emergently. If comorbidities exist, however, that cause slow bleeding, for example, peptic ulcer disease, menstruation, or kidney stones, the risks and benefits of performing surgery must be weighed thoughtfully to determine if surgery should be postponed until bleeding has stopped or blood counts return to normal.

Observe Patients not only Laboratory Results

Are patients symptomatic (tachycardic, short of breath with exertion, diaphoretic, or light headed), possibly indicative of an acute anemia? Are other nonspecific clues to chronic anemia displayed, such as complaints of being tired all the time, complaints of chest pain, increase in falls, poor eating and sleeping, increased irritability or confusion, bleeding gums, and pale or cool skin? Patients having one or more of these symptoms may indicate anemia and the need for further assessment.

Chronic anemias may be well tolerated by some patients; however, attempts should still be made to optimize a patient's hematologic status in preparation for surgery. This may mean, at times, not achieving the ideal "normal"' values but maximizing this patient's potential for a safe surgical course. The importance of questioning the accuracy of results when they do not seem to correspond with the patient "picture" is demonstrated in case study 2.

Case Study 2

A 59-year-old female patient presents to an emergency room by ambulance with multiple episodes of hematemesis and complaints of feeling weak and lightheaded. She has no prior history of peptic ulcer disease, no melena, and no heartburn or indigestion; is positive for arthritis; and is currently taking aspirin (650 mg per day) for hip and knee pain. Laboratory results indicate Hgb 5.4 and Hct 16%, which triggers an emergent call for gastrointestinal (GI) physician consult. The consult is completed quickly and an upper endoscopy is performed in the emergency room. No active bleeding is found.

What is a reasonable course of treatment in this situation? The patient was typed and cross-matched for transfusion at which time she expressed her request for nonblood medical management. This made the immediate response and follow-up of the on-call GI physician vital to ensure the safest outcome possible for this patient. Would you have done something differently? Likely few of us would have.

In this patient's case, abnormal critical laboratory results were rechecked and showed her actual Hgb and Hct results were 8.9 and 26%, respectively. She was admitted for observation and, although mildly symptomatic, never felt as though she were in imminent danger. She was alert and oriented and her vital signs remained within normal limits. The urgent response was appropriate based on the laboratory values. She was subsequently discharged home in stable condition. This case study demonstrates the need to confirm results while acting quickly to appropriately treat a potentially life-threatening condition.

Managing Anemia

Iron deficiency anemia is common and simply supplementing with iron and dietary changes often corrects the anemia. If expedience is indicated, intravenous (IV) iron has proved effective. In the authors' practice, iron sucrose (Venofer) has been well tolerated by a majority of patients. If oral iron is ordered, patient compliance should be evaluated, as often it is discontinued by patients because of GI side effects (nausea or constipation).

A newer oral therapy produced by Colorado Biolabs, heme iron polypeptide with or without folic acid (Proferrin and Proferrin Forte), also is being used and has proved advantages to other oral therapies. It is not altered by taking with food,[21] has reduced GI side effects comparable to IV iron,[22] and is highly absorbed.[23] Only the formula with folic acid (Proferrin Forte) requires a prescription.

In more severe anemias erythropoietin (Epogen or Procrit) or darbepoetin (Alfa Aranesp) perhaps is beneficial. They typically are given in conjunction with iron, unless patients have adequate iron stores. Although an initial response to erythropoietin/darbepoetin (EPO) can be seen within a week, it usually takes several weeks to see the full benefit. Elective surgeries should allow the necessary time for adequate response to this treatment as confirmed by laboratory test results. In emergent cases, initiating EPO treatment concurrently with other medical or surgical intervention facilitates maximum patient benefit. Unfortunately, despite its worldwide approval in the surgical setting beginning in 1993, acceptance of EPO therapy as an alternative to blood transfusion has been slow.[24]

Diet

Dietary measures that may be recommended to patients who are anemic to better prepare themselves for surgery may include increased intake of meat protein, almonds, leafy green vegetables, brown rice, peanut butter, beans, and dried fruits. Supplementation with oral iron, vitamin C, folic acid, and vitamin B complex also may improve red blood cells (RBCs) and health.

Thrombocytopenia

Low platelet counts might warrant use of IV immunoglobulin or oprelvekin (Neumega), which can stimulate platelet production, particularly in preparation for a procedure. IV immunoglobulin typically brings platelet counts to a safe level within 1 to 3 days. The effect, however, is temporary, and may last only as long as several weeks. It is used to treat idiopathic thrombocytopenia purpura,[25] other thrombocytopenic conditions, life-threatening bleeding, and in preparation for surgical procedures.

Oprelvekin is used for the short-term treatment of thrombocytopenia, and may take an average of 2 weeks to reach a safe platelet count. Labeled use is prophylaxis for or treatment of severe thrombocytopenia. Its purpose is to reduce the need for platelet transfusions after myelosuppressive chemotherapy in adult patients who have nonmyeloid malignancies and who are at high risk for severe thrombocytopenia. It also is used off label to increase platelet counts preoperatively and in select other medical conditions of severe thrombocytopenia.

MEDICATIONS TO CONTROL BLEEDING

Is it possible to avoid an invasive surgery or continued blood loss with the use of a medication? Coagulation factor VIIa (NovoSeven) currently has indications for treatment in hemophilia but its off-label use is rapidly growing and is greater than its indicated use in hemophilic patients.[26] It has been reported to control bleeding in other situations when conventional treatment has been unsuccessful, such as major trauma,[27,28] thrombocytopenia,[29] warfarin overdose,[30] obstetric bleeding,[31] and intracranial bleeding.[32]

Vitamin K may be another inexpensive and effective treatment in a bleeding situation. A patient's response to treatment is easily tracked to determine efficacy.

Where medical management is not an option or is not a sufficient treatment in itself, minimally invasive procedures may allow mitigating blood loss while treating patients.

PREOPERATIVE AUTOLOGOUS BLOOD DONATION—GOOD MEDICINE?

Studies show that preoperative autologous blood donation (PAD) may not prevent patients from receiving an allogeneic blood transfusion. In fact, 50% of patients who donate blood before surgery present with anemia on the day of surgery.[33] PAD did not optimize these patients for surgery. When considering risks associated with transfusion, it is important to remember that PAD is autologous banked blood. This means it may be subject to clerical errors similar to allogeneic blood[34] and does not, therefore, eliminate the risk for transmission of disease. Being a banked product, it also carries the risk for bacterial contamination and transfusion reactions, such as immunomodulation from leukocyte activation, depletion of nitrous oxide during storage, and changes in the structure of the red cell flexibility, making it incapable of efficiently delivering oxygen to the microcirculation.

INTRAOPERATIVE CONSIDERATIONS
Minimally Invasive Procedures

When complications are not encountered, minimally invasive options yield significantly less blood loss than open surgeries. There always is an associated risk for bleeding that needs to be addressed by converting to an open approach. This may delay treatment of the bleed and in the end cause greater blood loss. Surgeons must take all of these factors and comorbidities into consideration.

Endoscopy

Endoscopy may be used in conjunction with cautery, fibrin sealants, or other therapies to identify and control bleeding. Typically, patients recover quickly and are able to return home within a short period of time.

Cell tagging

Cell tagging is used to locate a source of bleeding, source of infection, or abnormal vascularities. Historically, surgeons have resorted to exploratory surgery, with its higher risk for bleeding, to identify the problem. This technology can minimize the need for more invasive procedures.

Interventional radiology/selective arterial embolization

Selective arterial embolization can be used to cut off blood supply to a tumor, organ, aneurism, or uterine fibroid or to quell postpartum hemorrhage.[35] Case studies 3 and 4 show examples of successful use of this procedure.

Case Study 3

A 76-year-old male patient arrives at the emergency room by ambulance with acute onset of sharp, constant left flank pain, followed by a bloody bowel movement. Flank pain is increased upon movement and palpation. Patient denies blood in urine or recent trauma. Patient is mildly hypertensive but otherwise vital signs are within normal limits. Patient does not appear pale, diaphoretic, or disoriented. There is a medical history of atrial fibrillation and recent history of ischemic cerebrovascular accident for which he was prescribed warfarin. International normalized ratio is 5.3 and initial Hgb level 13.4. CT scan shows a left renal cystic mass with hematoma. The patient is found in hemorrhagic shock secondary to intra-abdominal bleeding resulting from overcoagulation and renal mass. Patient is given fluid resuscitation and activated factor VII (to control bleeding) and taken to radiology where he has successful multiple embolizations of the left renal artery. The patient responds well to treatment and shortly thereafter returns home without further problems to await possible future removal of the embolized kidney.

Case Study 4

A 55-year-old female patient who has known chronic myelomonocytic leukemia presents to the hospital with increasing abdominal distention and shortness of breath. Patient has a history of progressive splenic enlargement, which has gone untreated because none of the physicians in her locality were willing to approach her care with the restriction on the use of blood or blood replacement therapy in her management. Being unaware that there were other options available, she and her family were resigned to a probable adverse outcome. Presenting laboratory results are as follows: WBC 25.8, Hgb 10.2, Hct 31%, and platelet count 38,000. CT scan shows massive splenomegaly with areas of possible early infarction of the spleen and increasing abdominal pain consistent with impending splenic rupture. Splenic artery embolization is completed by an interventional radiologist and 4 days later a nearly 8-pound spleen is removed. After splenectomy, platelet count rises to 40,000 and continues to rise until at discharge on day 14, patient's platelet count is 189,000 and Hgb and Hct are stable at 6.3 and 19%, respectively.

Selective arterial embolization has proved an underutilized, minimally invasive, effective option for treating many patients safely and avoiding transfusion.

Laparoscopic or robot-assisted laparoscopic surgery

Blood loss and complications typically are reduced in laparoscopic and robot-assisted laparoscopic surgeries versus open surgical approaches. Risk factors with both include unexpected bleeding and the need for conversion to an open procedure. Robot-assisted procedures, primarily because they are a new technology and a learning curve is involved, also often mean longer anesthesia times. The significant reduction in blood loss associated with robot-assisted laparoscopic radical prostatectomy (RALRP) versus open prostatectomy is well documented.[36,37] This blood loss reduction also was quantified in a study completed by Miller and colleagues[38] at the University of North Carolina, in which they found that RALRP reduced blood loss on average from 490 mL with open surgical techniques to 232 mL with robotic. In most published studies, complication rates in radical prostatectomy are 8%-20% in open surgeries and 4%–10% in robotic assisted surgery.[39] Similar results have been seen in cardiothoracic and gynecologic surgeries using laparoscopic and robot-assisted technology. Smaller incisions typically mean reduced recovery time, pain, and trauma.[40]

Surgical Techniques

Many of the surgical techniques pioneered in an effort to provide transfusion-free care have now become the standard of care. Surgeons recognize the need for meticulous surgical technique to maintain hemostasis, especially with increasing numbers of patients requesting treatment without the use of blood products. Constant awareness of patients' coagulative state can prevent unnecessary blood loss. Simple things can be implemented, such as positioning patients in a way that elevates the surgical site to reduce arterial pressure and facilitates venous drainage away from the surgical wound,[41] applying tourniquets or local vasoconstrictors to the surgical wound, and using topical hemostats. Anesthesia techniques, such as hypotensive anesthesia and maintaining normothermia, also play a vital role.

Surgical Equipment and Procedures

Hemostasis

Blood loss can be reduced by means of everything from older technologies, such as electrocautery and argon beam coagulation, to newer technology, such as fibrin sealants, and the Aquamantys System (Transcollation technology, Salient Surgical Technologies, Dover, New Hampshire [formerly TissueLink Medical]).

Blood salvage and autotransfusion

Blood can be salvaged preoperatively in the case of acute normovolemic hemodilution (ANH), intraoperatively with cell salvage, or postoperatively by means of wound drainage, and later reinfused into patients. These methods virtually remove the risk for transmission of foreign pathogens and allow patients to benefit from the oxygen-carrying capacity of their own blood cells.

Perioperative autologous cell salvage, also known as intraoperative autotransfusion, suctions all lost blood possible from the surgical wound and, in the case of moderate to severe blood loss, can separate, wash, and reinfuse the RBCs into patients.

ANH is used in cases with expected high-volume blood loss. Shortly after a patient's arrival to the operating room, several units of blood are diverted from the patient into blood bags, and the volume then is replaced with colloid or crystalloid solution. The diverted blood volume is kept anticoagulated in the operating room awaiting reinfusion. Volume loss during surgery remains approximately the same but contains fewer RBCs. When bleeding is controlled or at the end of surgery, the blood diverted preoperatively is reinfused. Because this process is completed at the patient's bedside, there is no storage or screening involved, costs are kept to a minimum, and the risk for human error is virtually eliminated, making this an advantageous procedure compared with PAD.[42] Although the risks for ANH are not quantified, they seem minimal.[43] Given the reported results of clinical trials completed to date, scientists are fairly confident that ANH does not pose a major risk for patients.

Diversion of blood from the surgical site

The heart-lung pump, or extracorporeal circulation, allows surgeons to perform open heart surgeries that otherwise are impossible. Among the risks associated with this procedure are increased bleeding risk, resulting from high volume anticoagulation and platelet damage, and inflammatory processes. Because of this, there is a new trend among cardiothoracic surgeons toward off-pump or beating heart coronary artery bypass grafting (CABG). Using this technique, cell damage that inherently occurs with use of the heart-lung pump is avoided, and less anticoagulant is needed, thereby reducing the bleeding risk and need for allogeneic transfusion. Off-pump CABG is not an option in all situations, such as valve replacement. Minimally invasive CABG is another emerging technique that ideally reduces the risk for bleeding, scarring, and infection but, as with other minimally invasive procedures, benefits must be weighed against risks and in the light of comorbidities.

Modified ultrafiltration[44] was introduced in the early 1990s as a technique to hemoconcentrate the residual blood in the extracorporeal circuit along with the patient's existing blood volume post cardiopulmonary bypass. It carried with it inherent risks, including hemodynamic instability, difficulty purging the entire extracorporeal circuit without redilution of the patient volume, and loss of residual blood that is left in the modified ultrafiltration system at its completion. The Hemobag (Global Blood Resources, Somers, Connecticut) is a modification of this system used by a perfusionist to accomplish hemoconcentration without the associated risks (described previously).

Many strategies have been discussed that can be used pre- and intraoperatively to facilitate a safer surgical experience for patients who refuse blood products. The care of patients who have returned to the floor after a successful surgery with no more than the expected blood loss, perhaps with drains in place, is discussed. What can nurses look for and implement in the postoperative phase to support patients through a safe and uneventful recovery period?

POSTOPERATIVE CONSIDERATIONS

A key to a safe and successful postoperative experience is monitoring patients and intervening early rather than adopting a wait-and-see attitude when there is some concern. Advocate for patients. Early intervention averts adverse medical events and crisis management. Trust professional instincts. Look at patients; listen to patients; if there is a negative trend in a patient's condition, act rather than wait. Advocating for patients may mean contacting an attending physician or specialist at times other than regular office hours. This may require persistence.

Have there been significant changes in the appearance of a wound, drainage, patient pain level, or vital signs that might indicate a decline in a patient's hematologic condition? Several aspects of caring for transfusion-free patients are discussed.

Wound Assessment

Monitor wound drainage: is it greater than expected for this type of procedure? Is the patient experiencing greater than normal swelling or discoloration of the wound site? Is the patient complaining of unmanaged pain? Swelling and pain may indicate internal bleeding. Are the laboratory results trending in a negative direction? Has the surgeon been made aware and have appropriate orders been received?

Is reinfusion of wound drainage an option for the patient? Depending on a particular hospital's policy, there typically is a 4- to 6-hour window to reinfuse wound drainage that has been collected into a sterile reservoir. Discuss this option with the physician and then with the patient. Some patients requesting nonblood management require that wound drainage devices be set up in a continuous circuit, meaning that the drain was placed and the line from the reservoir back to the patient IV was primed during surgery.

Supportive Measures—Diet and Exercise

Often underestimated is the importance of diet and exercise in healing and anemias. A high-protein diet promotes healing. Nutritional supplements, including vitamins C and B_{12}, folic acid, and iron, are necessary for healthy RBC production. This is especially important in patients who may be anemic. Adequate activity promotes an appropriate bone marrow response to increase RBC production and minimizes the risk for thrombophlebitis.

Phlebotomy

It is not uncommon to see patients return from surgery with laboratory tests ordered to be drawn anywhere from every few hours to once a day thereafter during their hospital stay. Are they truly necessary to provide quality health care to individuals? Or are patients jeopardized by removing vital resources that could be better used in the healing process? Dr. Howard Corwin, a respected leader in bloodless medicine strategies, chief of Critical Care Medicine and medical director of the intensive care setting at Dartmouth-Hitchcock Medical Center, concluded that patients who stay in an intensive care setting for more than a week often require a blood transfusion solely because of the volume of blood removed by phlebotomy.[45,46] Dr. Corwin's conclusions have been confirmed and are shared by other critical care providers. When dealing with a patient population in which blood transfusions are not an option, every drop of blood counts. It is imperative to modify phlebotomy practices. Limiting phlebotomy to necessary tests and using point-of-care devices, short-fill, or pediatric tubes can help to that end.

Vital Signs

Monitor vital signs closely, including oxygenation. Remember that if patients are anemic, even if their oxygen saturation seems adequate per pulse oximetry, they are likely not perfusing tissues adequately and could benefit from oxygen. If patients are not symptomatic (short of breath or lightheaded), this is a modality that often is overlooked.

Address hypertension immediately. It stands to reason that increased pressure causes patients to be more prone to bleeding.

Hydration

Monitor hydration. If patients are dehydrated, Hct, which indicates percentage of RBCs in the circulating volume, may seem adequate when patients actually are anemic. On the other end of the spectrum, patients who are fluid overloaded appear more anemic than they actually are.

Medications

If antiplatelets and anticoagulants are ordered, continue to closely monitor patients for signs of bleeding. Assess for warning signs, such as bleeding gums, IV sites, increased wound bleeding, or blood tinged urine.

Promptly addressing changes in patients' condition can facilitate their safe return home. In a bleeding or anemia situation, time is of the essence. Do not hesitate to report concerns to a physician. You just might save a life.

SUMMARY

An increasing number of patients and medical professionals are expressing an interest in bloodless medicine or blood conservation. Successful implementation of nonblood strategies and techniques has led to dramatic and impressive results. Each year more studies are published that indicate that the treatment methods held as standard for decades, almost religiously, may not be the safest and most appropriate approach in treating patients. The evidence consistently indicates that preventative measures to reduce bleeding and anemias and judicious use of blood products is simply the best medicine. Medical studies confirm that there are fewer infections, shorter hospital stays, and even reduced mortality when compared with those patients who receive blood transfusions.

A successful approach incorporates the collective efforts of a multifaceted team. Skilled physicians and surgeons play a key role on the successful team. They take the necessary precautions and time using procedures, pharmaceuticals, and medical technology to avoid the need for transfusions. Many physician-based organizations have been formed to educate and publish recommendations for improved practice in regard to blood use. The Society for the Advancement of Blood Management, Network for Advancement of Transfusion Alternatives, and Association of American Blood Banks are just a few such organizations.

Capable and compassionate nurses provide the best medical care possible within the parameters of patients' expressed and informed wishes. Nurses are the eyes and ears that can identify a trend and activate a prompt response to avert adverse medical outcomes. A supportive hospital administration upholds patient rights and provides appropriately equipped facilities and trained medical professionals as a center of excellence for patient care.

Regardless of the reasons patients make a choice to decline blood transfusions, safe and effective alternatives are available. The authors believe that transfusion-free medicine and blood conservation are the future of medicine and will continue to prove themselves the gold standard.

REFERENCES

1. Remmers PA, Speer AJ. Clinical strategies in the medical care of Jehovah's Witnesses. Am J Med 2006;119(12):1013–8.
2. Protecting the nation's blood supply from infectious agents: the need for new standards to meet new threats. Committee on Government Reform and Oversight; 1996.
3. Day M. Two week old blood no good for transfusion. New Scientist Web site. Available at: www.newscientist.com/article/dn13501-twoweekold-blood-no-good-for-transfusions.html. 2008; Accessed July 12, 2008.
4. Nowak R. Blood transfusions found to harm some patients. New Sci 2008;2653:8–9.
5. Vamvakas EC, Carven JH. Allogeneic blood transfusion, hospital charges, and length of hospitalization: a study of 487 consecutive patients undergoing colorectal cancer resection. Arch Pathol Lab Med 1998;122:145–51.
6. Hill GE, Frawley WH, Griffith KE, et al. Allogeneic blood transfusion increases the risk of postoperative bacterial infection: a meta-analysis. J Trauma 2003;54:908–14.
7. Blachman MA. Transfusion immunomodulation or TRIM: what does it mean clinically? Hematology 2005;10(Suppl):208–14.
8. Shander A, Hofmann A, Bombotz H, et al. Estimating the cost of blood: past, present, and future directions. Best Pract Res Clin Anaesthesiol 2007;21(2):271–89.
9. American Association of Blood Banks, America's Blood Centers, American Red Cross. Circular of information for the use of human blood and blood components. Bethesda (MD): American Association of Blood Banks; 2002. p. 15.
10. Farmer S, Webb D. Your body, your choice. Singapore: Media Masters; 2000. p. 72–4.
11. Smith ML. Ethical perspectives on Jehovah's Witnesses' refusal of blood. Cleve Clin J Med 1997;64(9):475–81.
12. Appelbaum PS, Roth LH. Patients who refuse treatment in medical hospitals. J Am Med Assoc 1983; 250:1296–301.
13. Mill JS. On liberty. In: Adler MJ, editor, Great books of the western world, vol. 43. Chicago, IL: Encylopedia Brittanica, Inc.; 1952. p. 273.
14. Murphy G, Reeves B, Rogers C, et al. Increased mortality, postoperative morbidity, and cost after red blood cell transfusion in patients having cardiac surgery. Circulation 2007;116(22):2544–52.
15. Goodnough LT, Shander A, Brecher ME. Transfusion medicine: looking towards the future. Lancet 2003; 361s:161–9.
16. Blumberg N. Transfusion-alternative strategies. Brooklyn (NY): Watchtower Bible and Tract Society of New York, Inc.; 2004.
17. Shorr A, Jackson W, Kelly K, et al. Transfusion practice and blood stream infections in critically ill patients. Chest 2005;127:1722–8.

18. Fauci A, Braunwald E, Isselbacher K, et al. Transfusion biology and therapy. Harrison's principles of internal medicine. 14th edition. New York: McGraw-Hill; 1998:721(Table 115-3).

19. Rosenblatt M, Mindel J. Spontaneous hyphema associated with ingestion of Ginkgo biloba extract. N Engl J Med 1997;336:1108.

20. Cupp MJ. Herbal remedies: adverse effects and drug interactions. Am Fam Physician 1999;59:1239–44.

21. Uzel C, Conrad ME, Umbreit JN. Absorption of heme iron. Semin Hematol 1998;35:27–34.

22. Nissenson A, Berns J, Sakiewicz P, et al. Clinical evaluation of heme iron polypeptide: sustaining a response to rHuEPO in hemodialysis patients. Am J Kidney Dis 2003;42(2):325–30.

23. Seligman P, Moore G, Schleicher R. Clinical studies of HIP: an oral heme-iron product. Nutr Res 2000; 20(9):1279–86.

24. Goodnough LT, Monk TG, Andriole GL. Erythropoietin therapy. N Engl J Med 1997;336:933–8.

25. George JN, Woolf SH, Raskob GE, et al. Idiopathic thrombocytopenic purpura: a practice guideline developed by explicit methods for the American Society of Hematology. Blood 1996;88(1):3–40.

26. De Gasperi A. Intraoperative use of recombinant activated factor VII (r-FVIIa). Minerva Anesthesiol 2006; 72:489–94.

27. Chiara O, Cimbanassi S, Brioschi PR, et al. Treatment of critical bleeding in trauma patients. Minerva Anesthesiol 2006;72:383–7.

28. Gowers CJD, Parr MJA. Recombinant activated factor VIIa use in massive transfusion and coagulopathy unresponsive to conventional therapy. Anaesth Intensive Care 2005;33:196–200.

29. Goodnough LT. Experiences with recombinant human factor VIIa in patients with thrombocytopenia. Semin Hematol 2004;41(1 Suppl. 1):25–9.

30. Lin J, Hanigan WC, Tarantino M, et al. The use of recombinant activated factor VII to reverse warfarin-induced anticoagulation in patients with hemorrhages in the central nervous system: preliminary findings. J Neurosurg 2003;98:737–40.

31. Heilmann L, Wild C, Hojnacki B, et al. Successful treatment of life-threatening bleeding after cesarean section with recombinant activated factor VII. Clin Appl Thromb Hemost 2006;12:227–9.

32. Karadimov D, Krassimir B, Nachkov Y, et al. Use of activated recombinant factor VII (NovoSeven) during neurosurgery. J Neurosurg Anesthesiol 2003;15:330–2.

33. Forgie M, Wells P, Laupacis A, et al. Preoperative autologous donation decreased allogeneic transfusion but increases exposure to all red cell transfusion: results of a meta analysis. International Study of Perioperative Transfusion (ISPOT) Investigators. Arch Intern Med 1998;158:610–6.

34. Mackey J, Lipton KS. Association Bulletin 95-4, AABB position on testing of autologous units. Bethesda, MD: American Association of Blood Banks; 1995.

35. Roman AS, Rebarber A. Seven ways to control postpartum hemorrhage. Contemp Ob Gyn 2003;48(3): 34–53.

36. Tewari A, Srivasatava A, Menon M, et al. A prospective comparison of radical retropubic and robot-assisted prostatectomy: experience in one institution. BJU Int 2003;92:205–10.

37. Ahlering TE, Woo D, Eichel L, et al. Robot assisted versus open prostatectomy: a comparison of one surgeon's outcomes. Urology 2004;63:819–22.

38. Miller J, Smith A, Kouba E, et-al. Prospective evaluation of short-term impact and recovery of health related quality of life in men undergoing robotic assisted laparoscopic radical prostatectomy versus open radical prostatectomy, submitted for publication.

39. Basillotte J, Ahlering TE, Skarecky DW, et al. Laparoscopic radical prostatectomy: review and assessment of an emerging technique. Surg Endosc 2004;18:1694–711.

40. Intuitive Surgical Web site. 2005. Available at: www.intuitivesurgical.com/patientresources/conditions/thoracic/index.aspx. [Accessed 12, July 2008].

41. Schneeberger AG, Schulz RF, Ganz R. Blood loss in total hip arthroplasty. Lateral position combined with preservation of the capsule versus supine position combined with capsulectomy. Arch Orthop Trauma Surg 1998;117(1–2):47–9.

42. Monk TG, Goodnough LT, Birkmeyer JD, et al. Acute normovolemic hemodilution is a cost-effective alternative to preoperative autologous blood donation by patients undergoing radical retropubic prostatectomy. Transfusion 1995;35:559–65.

43. Shander A, Rijhwani TS. Acute normovolemic hemodilution. Transfusion 2004;44(Suppl 12):26S–34S.

44. Moskowitz D, Klein J, Shander A, et al. Use of the hemobag for modified ultrafiltration in a Jehovah's Witness patient undergoing cardiac surgery. JECT 2006;38:265–70.

45. Corwin H, Parsonnet K, Gettinger A. RBC transfusion in the ICU is there a reason? Chest 1995;108: 767–71.

46. Chant C, Wilson G, Friedrich JO. Anemia, transfusion, and phlebotomy practices in critically ill patients with prolonged ICU length of stay: a cohort study. Crit Care 2006;10(5):R140.

Perioperative Patient Safety and Procedural Sedation

Jan Odom-Forren, MS, RN, CPAN, FAAN*

KEYWORDS

- Patient safety • Procedural sedation
- Sedation and analgesia • Sedation risk factors
- Nurse-administered propofol sedation
- Safe sedation practice

The concept of patient safety was brought to the forefront in 1999 when the Institute of Medicine published *To Err is Human: Building a Safer Health System*.[1] The authors of the report focused on the impact of medical or health care errors occurring with or to patients and delineated patient safety as a priority for the health care community. The report pointed out that error was the property of a system of care as opposed to individual health care providers and that those systems should provide well-designed processes of care that result in prevention, recognition, and early recovery from errors to ensure that patients remain safe and unharmed.[2]

The use of sedation administered by nonanesthesia providers for procedures has increased exponentially over the past decade. Procedural sedation is performed in the perioperative environment and in nonsurgical environments such as the endoscopy suite, the cardiac catheterization laboratory, the labor and delivery suite, physician offices, emergency departments, and dental offices. This use of procedural or nurse-monitored sedation has partially been driven by economic factors, with some insurance companies not wanting to pay anesthesia providers for routine procedures, and by the need to move patients quickly through the procedural area—a more difficult process when scheduling anesthesia.[3]

The safety of the patient is the primary concern for perioperative nurses who are involved in administering sedation or in monitoring the patient who has received procedural sedation.[4] Moderate sedation is safe but has potential adverse reactions such as hypoxemia, apnea, hypotension, airway obstruction, and cardiopulmonary arrest.[5,6] As a member of the Dartmouth Summit stated, "the side effects of the procedure can traumatize you; the side effects of the sedation can kill you".[7] The nurse, however, cannot guarantee the safety of the patient alone or in a silo. Patient safety is the responsibility of every person on the perioperative team and relies on an effective sedation delivery system to keep the patient from harm.

SEDATION ISSUES RELATING TO PATIENT SAFETY
Sedation on a Continuum

Sedation falls on a continuum from minimal sedation to deep sedation. Typically, nurse-monitored sedation falls under the definition of moderate sedation. Minimal sedation is used to decrease anxiety but does not affect the patient's respiratory or cardiovascular functions; however, the patient is under the influence of the medication and should be treated as such. The patient receiving moderate sedation should be able to maintain respirations without significant cardiovascular changes. With this type of sedation, the patient is able to respond to verbal or mild tactile stimulation. The risk for complications increases as the patient moves on the continuum from minimal to moderate sedation. The patient who is receiving moderate sedation has the potential to move into deep sedation and thus become at higher risk for complications. A patient receiving deep sedation should respond

University of Kentucky, Lexington, KY, USA
* 800 Edenwood Circle, Louisville, KY 40243, USA
E-mail address: jodom29373@aol.com

Perioperative Nursing Clinics 3 (2008) 355–366
doi:10.1016/j.cpen.2008.08.010

to repeated or painful stimulation and is at risk for respiratory compromise, although cardiovascular status is usually preserved. If the patient receiving sedation is unresponsive, that patient is receiving general anesthesia with risk for respiratory compromise, cardiac compromise, or both.[6,8,9] The further the patient moves on the continuum, the greater the risk for the patient (**Table 1**).

The nurse who is monitoring a patient during procedural sedation must be able to rescue a patient who inadvertently moves from one level of sedation to the next level of sedation. Therefore, the nurse monitoring the patient who is receiving moderate sedation should be prepared to rescue the patient who moves into deep sedation, and the nurse monitoring the patient during deep sedation must be prepared to rescue a patient who has respiratory or cardiovascular compromise and who has moved on the continuum into general anesthesia.

Adverse Reactions

Respiratory depression is the most common adverse reaction to procedural sedation. One panel discussing the risks of sedation noted that sedation complications are related to *underuse* complications that cause patients to suffer pain and stress, *overuse* complications that can result in respiratory depression or apnea, or *misuse* complications that involve errors in drug administration such as accidentally giving sufentanil instead of fentanyl.[7] Cote and colleagues[10] studied adverse sedation events in pediatric patients. In this critical incident analysis, there were 60 events that resulted in death or permanent central nervous system injury. Respiratory depression was the first event in 80% of the patients. Poor outcome was associated with inadequate resuscitation, inadequate monitoring, inadequate initial evaluation, and inadequate recovery phase.

In a report of adverse events during pediatric sedation and anesthesia outside the operating room, 26 institutions submitted data on 30,037 patients for a period of 17 months. Serious adverse events were rare, with no deaths and cardiopulmonary resuscitation being required only once. Less serious events occurred, such as oxygen desaturation below 90% for more than 30 seconds (157 times per 10,000 sedations), unexpected apnea (24 times per 10,000 sedations), and vomiting (47.2 per 10,000 sedations). Even with a low incidence of serious adverse reactions to pediatric sedation, the number of events that had potential to harm was significant, occurring once every 89 sedations.[11] Because events with the potential to compromise patient safety are so common, it is imperative that personnel involved in sedation are competent to manage an airway obstruction, emesis, hypoventilation, and apnea.[12]

Adverse reactions to sedation are an international problem. From a questionnaire sent to nonanesthesia providers to assess sedation practices in Ireland, Fanning[13] found that 22% of respondents reported events ranging from respiratory depression, hypoxia, loss of consciousness, prolonged sedation, and nausea and vomiting. Two events required the presence of an anesthesia provider.[13] Sedation was the cause of most complications that occurred in a study conducted in Germany to determine complications in outpatient gastrointestinal endoscopy patients.[14]

In 121 monitored anesthesia care cases pulled from the American Society of Anesthesiologists (ASA) Closed Claims database (1990–2002), the severity of complications was similar to that found with general anesthesia.[15] Twenty-one percent of the claims were due to respiratory depression secondary to the sedative medications. These events were associated with older age ($\geq$70 years), ASA physical status III and IV, and obesity. Propofol or benzodiazepines used alone were associated

---

Table 1
Levels of sedation

Function	Level of Sedation			
	Minimal	Moderate	Deep	General Anesthesia
Responsiveness	Normal response to verbal stimulation	Purposeful response to light stimulation	Purposeful response to pain stimulation	Unarousable, even to painful stimulation
Airway	Unaffected	No intervention	Possible intervention	Probable intervention
Ventilation	Unaffected	Adequate	May be inadequate	Often inadequate
Cardiovascular	Unaffected	Usually maintained	Usually maintained	May be impaired

Data from Refs.[5–7]

with oversedation in 9% of the patients. Propofol with the use of another medication was responsible for 50% of the oversedation.[15] This information about patients receiving monitored anesthesia care can be assumed to also apply to patients receiving sedation and analgesia from nonanesthesia providers.

The low percentages of serious complications such as aspiration or hypoxia with resulting neurologic impairment or death require that larger studies be undertaken than have been conducted to date. Surrogate markers are typically used in studies to determine the potential for serious adverse reactions. A surrogate marker commonly used in sedation studies is respiratory depression, with an operational definition for the study such as apnea longer than 30 seconds or oxygen saturation below 90%. The occurrence of cardiopulmonary complications is used as a surrogate marker of the risk for occurrence of a significant adverse event.[5] Studies conducted with surrogate markers are able to use lower numbers of patients but have unclear clinical significance.[5,16] In summary, although the severe complication rates are low for procedural sedation, failure to recognize or immediately treat these patients can lead to morbidity or even death. Of great importance are patient risk assessment and rescue capabilities.[11]

Patient Risk Factors

Preprocedure assessment and identification of high-risk patients is the key to the prevention or successful management of sedation-related events.[17] Patients at high risk for complications should be evaluated during the preprocedure assessment for appropriateness of nurse-monitored sedation (**Table 2**).[6,17] Patients at risk for a difficult airway are important to identify because respiratory complications are commonly associated with sedation. Risk factors associated with a difficult airway include a history of problems with anesthesia or sedation, advanced rheumatoid arthritis, chromosomal abnormalities (eg, trisomy 21), and stridor, snoring, or sleep apnea.[6,18]

Use of Propofol for Sedation

The use of propofol by nonanesthesia providers in sedation and analgesia has been fraught with controversy.[4,8] The advantages of propofol (over benzodiazepines) include less nausea, more rapid onset, and shorter duration of action, facilitating faster recovery and discharge.[4,19–21] Zed and colleagues[22] evaluated the efficacy, safety, and patient satisfaction with the use of propofol for procedural sedation for 113 patients in the emergency department. One patient experienced vomiting, 0 experienced apnea, 9 experienced hypotension, and 7 felt pain on injection. All patients and most physicians were satisfied with the use of propofol. The investigators concluded that as part of a standardized protocol, propofol appears to be safe and effective, with high patient and physician satisfaction.[22] In three other studies that were conducted using

Table 2
Patients at high risk for sedation-related complications

Risk Factor	Intervention
Presence of airway abnormalities	Evaluate airway before sedation Evaluate for presence of sleep apnea
ASA classification status of III or greater	Evaluate a class III patient on an individual basis Consult with anesthesia provider for classes IV or V
Chronic obstructive pulmonary disease	Administer bronchodilators before procedure Titrate sedatives in small increments
Obesity	Pretreat with oral H_2 antagonist Titrate sedatives in small increments
Coronary artery disease	Prevent over- or undersedation Allow routine cardiac medications to be taken on day of procedure Administer supplemental oxygen
Chronic renal failure	Avoid long-acting opioids Administer small incremental doses of sedatives
Drug addiction	Use short-acting sedatives with incremental dosing Avoid use of reversal agents
Extremes of age (pediatric and elderly)	Administer individual and incremental dosing

Data from Refs. [6,17,18,49]

nurse-administered propofol sedation (NAPS) with a total of 11,000 patients in the gastrointestinal setting, the investigators found no major complications.[23–25] In an article from a university setting where NAPS is used on a regular basis, Overley and Rex[26] discussed the use of NAPS as cost-effective and satisfying for physicians and nurses. In one study of 33,743 endoscopic procedures using NAPS,[27] no cases of endotracheal intubation, death, neurologic sequelae, or other permanent injury occurred. Temporary bag-mask ventilation was required by 49 patients. The three centers with a training program conducted by anesthesiologists had a center-specific rate of respiratory events from 9 per 10,000 to 19 per 10,000.[27]

Opponents of the use of NAPS point out that the good outcomes of these studies conceal the risks with the use of propofol. Those risks include the tendency to attain deep sedation or even general anesthesia on the sedation continuum, with the resulting problems of airway obstruction and apnea. No reversal agent for propofol is available when these events occur.[4] Anesthesia providers are quick to note that the absence of morbidity or mortality in a smaller sample of patients should be moderated by the fact that morbidity and mortality for healthy patients undergoing anesthesia is only 1 in 300,000.[28] Vargo,[5] who believes that the safety and efficacy of propofol for use in sedation has been established, goes on to state that the current data in randomized controlled trials do not sufficiently answer the question of its safety compared with standard sedation and analgesia.

The jury is out on the widespread use of propofol for sedation until regulatory agencies, third-party payers, and professional societies come to the same conclusion about propofol's safety. One concern related to nurse-monitored sedation includes propofol's strict product labeling as an anesthetic agent to be used by persons trained in the administration of general anesthesia.[3] State Boards of Nursing have varying positions regarding the use of propofol administered by nurses, with some boards (eg, Indiana) stating that it is within the scope of nursing practice for a competent and educated nurse to administer propofol for sedation and others (eg, Florida) stating that is not within the scope of practice for a registered nurse to administer propofol.[8] If a perioperative nurse is asked to administer propofol for sedation, the nurse would need to assure that the State Board of Nursing in that particular state did not have a position statement denoting that propofol was not within the scope of practice for a registered nurse. The health care facility should also have a strict education program that not only determines cognitive knowledge but also uses mentoring to determine competence.

A new drug, fospropofol sodium, is presently undergoing studies. Fospropofol is a water-soluble prodrug of propofol and will be used by determining a weight-based bolus.[5] It is unknown whether the increased plasma half-life will mean prolonged recovery, but it is hoped that the drug will be able to maintain a patient at the level of moderate sedation. Therefore, fospropofol would require a product label specifying the drug not as an anesthetic agent but as a sedative for administration by nonanesthesia providers. For short-duration procedures, it is possible that patients may require only a single dose.[29]

Guidelines for the ASA and the American Society for Gastrointestinal Endoscopy (ASGE) have specific criteria for monitoring patients who are under deep sedation, including a committed, qualified practitioner administering the sedation and the evaluation of ventilatory function with consideration of capnography.[6,29] The ASA and the ASGE have determined components of a training program for any health care facility that uses NAPS with resultant deep sedation. The ASGE includes an initial phase of training, including didactic material that discusses the sedative agents to be used, contraindications for specific agents, and certification in advanced cardiac life support or the equivalent. Other components of the ASGE program include a written test on didactic material, airway assessment, observation, and administration under supervision.[30] Contraindications to propofol administration by nonanesthesia providers at Indiana University where NAPS is widespread include increased aspiration risk (eg, acute upper gastrointestinal bleeding, achalasia, delayed gastric emptying, bowel obstruction); difficult airways (eg, sleep apnea requiring continuous positive airway pressure, marked obesity, abnormal airway assessment); extreme comorbidities; and allergy to propofol (or to eggs or soybeans).[30] The ASA has developed criteria that address the safe use of propofol when used by nonanesthesiologists (**Box 1**).

VanNatta and Rex[31] conducted a randomized clinical trial to compare recovery time and patient satisfaction with propofol administered alone titrated to deep sedation versus propofol plus fentanyl, propofol plus midazolam, or propofol plus a combination of midazolam and fentanyl titrated to moderate sedation in 200 outpatients undergoing colonoscopy. Patients who received a combination regimen were discharged more quickly. There were no significant differences in pain or satisfaction among the groups. This randomized controlled trial was the first to titrate propofol to

Box 1
Safe use of propofol
Responsible physician
Must have education and training to manage complications
Must be proficient in airway management
Must have advanced cardiac life support training
Must understand pharmacology of drugs
Practitioner administering propofol
Must have education and training to identify and manage airway and cardiovascular changes of patient who enters state of general anesthesia
Must have ability to assist in management of complications
Must be present throughout procedure, with no other responsibilities other than monitoring patient
Must monitor patient, assessing level of consciousness, ventilation, oxygen saturation, heart rate, and blood pressure, with monitoring of exhaled carbon dioxide when possible
Must identify early signs of hypotension, bradycardia, apnea, airway obstruction, oxygen desaturation
Must have age-appropriate equipment immediately available
Must not be involved in conduct of surgical/diagnostic procedure
From Odom-Forren J. The evolution of nurse monitored sedation. J Perianesth Nurs 2005;20:395; with permission.

moderate sedation in a combination therapy. The investigators stated that recognition among anesthesia providers of propofol as an agent that can be used for moderate sedation would be helpful in gaining acceptance of use by nonanesthesia personnel. The investigators also noted the importance of a defined training protocol, even when propofol is used for moderate sedation.

Mandel and colleagues[32] conducted a randomized controlled trial that compared two groups of patients using midazolam plus fentanyl or propofol plus remifentanil delivered by way of patient-controlled sedation (PCS). The patients who received propofol plus remifentanil recovered significantly faster than the group who received midazolam plus fentanyl. In the group administered propofol plus remifentanil, however, two patients required intervention by an anesthesiologist due to the

safety end point that was designed for the study of arterial desaturation below 85% for 60 seconds. The investigators stated that those who use this form of sedation must be prepared to administer resuscitative efforts immediately.

Computer-assisted personalized sedation (CAPS) is a method whereby continuous physiologic monitoring is combined with delivery of propofol sedation with the assistance of a computer interface and software. Twenty-four subjects were included in the stage I trial to assess the safeguard software. One subject experienced oxygen saturation below 90% and 7 subjects experienced apnea longer than 30 seconds. All 8 responded to automated device actions without intervention by an anesthesiologist. This initial study of an investigational device showed the viability of this technology to deliver propofol sedation to patients in the endoscopy suite.[33]

The importance of propofol and its relation to patient safety for the perioperative patient is its ability to move the patient quickly to deep sedation, with the resulting risk of respiratory compromise. To decrease those risks, studies have been conducted to assess for dosages of propofol that can be titrated to moderate sedation, new drugs are under development, and other methods of delivery systems (eg, PCS and CAPS) are in process to determine whether those methods would be safer for the patient.

SAFE SEDATION PRACTICE

In discussing vital issues that would decrease the harm associated with pediatric sedation, an expert panel identified the following priorities: the characterization of existing sedation care strategies across specialties, with data collected from multiple institutions; the proactive identification of hazards and vulnerabilities; improved sedation provider and team training with core competencies; systems research; and a patient-centered focus.[7] Performing safe and effective sedation involves several aspects of sedation, including (1) the persons administering the sedation, (2) the educational processes involved, (3) the environment in which the sedation is conducted, (4) patient-specific information processes, and (5) guidelines and protocols of the institution.

Qualified Individuals

The Joint Commission (TJC) requires that "qualified individuals" who administer sedation must possess education, training, and experience in evaluating patients before moderate or deep sedation, in rescuing patients who slip into a deeper level of sedation, and in managing a compromised airway or cardiovascular system during a procedure.[9] It is essential that those involved in procedural sedation have precompiled and practiced plans for respiratory events.[7] Examples of precompiled responses are basic life support and advanced cardiac life support. Panel members during one summit stated, "any failure to rescue is a marker for a flawed sedation care system that has not trained providers adequately."[7] One possible solution for hands-on rescue management is the use of human simulators. Simulators can re-create thousands of common or unusual events that clinicians learn to manage. Shavit and others[34] conducted a prospective, observational study in two university teaching hospitals in Israel to evaluate the impact of simulation-based education on patient safety during procedural sedation. Nonanesthesiologists who had training in simulation-based education were compared with those who did not receive the simulator-based education. A nine-criteria Sedation Safety Tool was used for evaluation. Significant differences in performance related to patient safety were found between the two groups of non-anesthesiologists. The researchers believed that the patient safety training was the reason for the superior performance of the physicians who had received the training and recommend simulation-based training in sedation safety for all nonanesthesiologists who practice pediatric procedural sedation. Knowing that death and failure to rescue have been determined as more frequent when care was not delivered by an anesthesia provider is impetus to determine the education necessary to provide safety for patients undergoing nurse-monitored procedural sedation.[35]

Box 2
Recommended airway management competencies

Basic airway assessment

Oral cavity inspection

Mallampati classification

Presence of a patent airway

Monitoring of the rate, depth, and general quality of respiratory effort

Pulse oximetry

Basic use and monitoring

Troubleshooting

Basic airway management

Airway maneuvers

Lateral head lift

Chin lift/support

Jaw thrust

Airway adjuncts

Nasal airway insertion

Oral airway insertion

Endotracheal tube insertion

Oxygen delivery devices

Advanced airway management

Use of a positive pressure ventilation device

Establishment of an airway by way of intubation

From Hooper V. Competence in patient management. In: Odom-Forren J, Watson D. Practical guide to moderate sedation/analgesia. 2nd edition. St. Louis (MO): Elsevier Mosby; 2005. p. 151; with permission.

Education and Competence

Competence involves skill, knowledge, action, and critical thinking. Individualized competency-based practice in the sedation environment develops as a result of education, professional literature, and practice.[36] Competencies of all sedation providers should include knowledge of medication administration and interaction, skill in airway management, and competence in dysrhythmia recognition and management (**Box 2**).[6,29,37] All health care providers who perform or monitor the patient undergoing procedural sedation should complete an educational program that includes competencies. Nonanesthesiologist physician providers should also provide evidence of competency. It is unfortunate that credentialing does not always relate to competency and is based on a professional title instead of demonstrated competency in skills needed.[7] Patient safety requires that the nurse providing the sedation recognize any problem, identify the cause, and take immediate and appropriate action to resuscitate the patient and rescue the patient from harm.[7]

Sedation Environment

TJC requires that health care facilities address the appropriate equipment for care, resuscitation, and monitoring of vital signs.[9] It is fortunate that serious adverse reactions do not occur on a routine basis. Therefore, current recommendations for monitoring the patient during sedation are based on surrogate markers (softer outcomes) such as transient hypoxemia or on expert opinion.[5] Pulse oximetry and capnography are objective physiologic measures. The relationship of these monitors to subsequent clinical interventions and effect of those interventions needs to be determined.[16]

Pulse oximetry, used to assess oxygenation, is an adjunct to clinical assessment for detecting hypoxemia. Pulse oximetry provides a noninvasive measure of the arterial hemoglobin oxygen saturation. Oxygen saturation occurs in direct proportion to the partial pressure of oxygen and provides an early indication of emergent hypoxemia.[8]

The use of pulse oximetry during sedation procedures has not been linked to a reduction in risk for cardiopulmonary complications.[5] Despite the lack of data linking pulse oximetry to fewer complications, however, nursing and physician organizations (eg, ASA, ASGE, Association of peri-Operative Registered Nurses, American Society of PeriAnesthesia Nurses, Society of Gastroenterology Nurses and Associates) guidelines require the use of pulse oximetry for all cases and suggest availability of supplemental oxygen.[5,6,29,37–39] The use of pulse oximetry is required by these guidelines based on studies that have identified respiratory depression with resulting hypoxemia as the precipitating factor in adverse events for adult and pediatric patients.[5] Monitoring oxygenation by use of a pulse oximeter is not a replacement for monitoring ventilatory function.[6,8]

Ventilatory function should be assessed apart from the use of pulse oximetry. Ventilatory function can be assessed by observing depth and rate of respirations or more accurately by auscultation of breath sounds.[8] Capnography measures ventilation (end-tidal carbon dioxide [CO_2]) by determining the amount of CO_2 in every breath and provides a graphic representation of exhaled CO_2 levels with a tracing called a capnogram.[8] The advantage of capnography is that it is a real-time display of the patient's ventilatory status and reflects apnea immediately. In one study of 80 patients undergoing colonoscopy procedures, researchers randomized patients into two groups: one group received supplemental oxygen and the other did not receive supplemental oxygen. Respiratory activity was monitored with a pretracheal stethoscope and capnography, and the staff was blinded to end-tidal CO_2 data. The investigators not only discovered that supplemental oxygen did not prevent apnea but also found that more patients who had apnea in the supplemental oxygen group went undetected by caregivers and received sedation following an apneic episode.[40] Vargo and colleagues[41] found that capnography was an excellent indicator of respiratory rate compared with auscultation. Of 54 episodes of apnea or disordered respiration occurring in 28 patients, only 50% of the episodes were detected by pulse oximetry. More important, no episode was detected by visual assessment.

Soto and colleagues[42] studied the use of capnography to determine whether it accurately detected apnea during monitored anesthesia care. In the study, 26% of 39 patients developed apnea of at least 20 seconds. These episodes were undetected by the anesthesia provider but were reliably detected by capnography and respiratory plethysmography, with no difference in detection rates between the two methods. Lightdale and others[43] published the first randomized controlled trial of capnography in pediatric patients undergoing endoscopy procedures during moderate sedation. The researchers sought to discover whether intervention based on capnographic evidence of alveolar hypoventilation would reduce the incidence of hypoxemia in these patients. Hypoventilation was defined as a pulse oximetry value of less than 95% for more than 5 seconds. In the control group, the sedation team was notified when alveolar hypoventilation lasted longer than 60 seconds. In the intervention group, the sedation team was notified when hypoventilation lasted longer than 15 seconds. When notified, the team would stimulate the patient by repositioning the patient's head and encouraging deep breaths. Patients in the intervention group were significantly less likely to experience hypoxemia compared with the control group. The researchers concluded that the use of capnography during moderate sedation decreased the incidence of arterial desaturation.[43]

Evidence that capnography is of assistance in the prevention of hypoventilation with a resulting decrease in hypoxemia is accumulating. At the present time, guidelines advocate the use of capnography any time a patient undergoes deep sedation.[6,29] It remains to be seen whether guidelines in the future will require monitoring of end-tidal CO_2 during moderate sedation. More research is needed to determine the clinical relevance and relationship to clinical interventions.[16]

Even with insufficient evidence to link hemodynamic monitoring to lack of complications, hemodynamic assessment is required because early detection of hemodynamic changes can result in early intervention, thus preventing a significant adverse event.[5] It is of interest that some organizational guidelines require the use of ECG monitoring on all patients receiving sedation,[37,38] whereas other organizations require the use of ECG monitoring on those receiving deep sedation or who have significant cardiopulmonary disease.[6,29,39] At a minimum, ECG monitoring should be considered when deep sedation is anticipated and in patients who have significant cardiac or pulmonary disease.[6,29,39]

The nurse involved in moderate sedation should have immediate access to suction equipment, supplemental oxygen, airway equipment including oral and nasal airways and a bag-mask device, reversal agents to counteract the affects of the benzodiazepines or opioids, and an emergency cart with a defibrillator. Alarms need to be set on monitors and all equipment needs to be in working order.

Patient-Specific Information

The patient should receive a procedure-specific history and physical examination. The primary purpose of a preprocedure nursing assessment is to gain baseline health information and to determine whether the patient has any illnesses or conditions that might preclude nurse-monitored sedation.[8] The history should include the medical diagnoses, any past experiences with sedation or anesthesia, current medications and herbals taken by the patient, and allergies (including medication and latex).

The physical evaluation by the monitoring registered nurse includes an assessment of the heart and lungs and an evaluation of the airway. Physical assessment includes baseline vital signs, height, weight, age, and oxygen saturation. The airway may be assessed using the Mallampati technique, which can be used to determine possible intubation difficulty.[44] The patient should be in a sitting position and directed to open the mouth as wide as possible. When the tongue is protruded, the faucial pillars and uvula should be visible. When the faucial pillars, soft palate, and uvula are not visible, the physician should be notified to determine the appropriate plan of action. Some facilities use a simple technique of observing for craniofacial abnormalities, asking the patient to stick out the tongue, open the mouth, and flex the neck to determine the potential for a difficult airway (**Box 3**).[8] An appropriate preprocedure assessment can decrease the risk of adverse outcomes and increase patient safety for patients receiving sedation.[6]

During the procedure, the patient should be monitored on an ongoing basis, with vital signs and oxygen saturation documented at least every 5 minutes. Any adverse reactions should be documented, and the nurse monitoring the patient should be alert to any changes in the patient's condition and immediately communicate that information to the provider. The level of consciousness should be assessed and the medication titrated in increments until the desired level is achieved.[8] Back-up personnel who are experts in airway management should be available in the event of a crisis. This availability is typically not as much of a problem in the perioperative area of the hospital as it is in non–operating room environments. When sedation is administered at night or during a weekend, however, help should be as easy to obtain as during busy times of the week.

The same monitoring parameters used during the procedure are used for postprocedure monitoring, with documentation at least every 15 minutes. Immediately after the procedure, the patient is at risk for respiratory depression because noxious stimuli have been removed, and the patient is allowed to rest without interference. The patient who received moderate sedation should be discharged using objective discharge criteria. An important aspect of discharge to keep the patient safe is to assure that a responsible adult escort is present to assist the patient home and care for the patient after discharge. Even patients who have received minimal sedation with the use of oral sedative agents should have a confirmed escort and the patient advised not to drive, make important decisions, or consume alcohol for at least 24 hours after the procedure.[45] Chung and Assmann[46] conducted a case review of litigations after ambulatory surgery that spanned a 10-year period. There were three malpractice cases of car accidents identified in patients who did not have an escort. In one case, the patient who was scheduled for a dilation and curettage under local anesthesia received lorazepam (1 mg orally) for antianxiety. The patient refused an offer for a ride home by a friend who worked in the post anesthesia care unit and drove herself home. On the drive home, she had a car accident, incurring serious injury, and sued the gynecologist and preoperative nurse who gave her the medication. The gynecologist and preoperative nurse were found negligent for allowing the patient to drive herself home. The injured parties in the second car also sued and were compensated. The investigators go on to state, "patients require escorts to go home regardless of the type of anesthesia."[46] Safe patient care requires that the caregiver cancel the case, admit the patient, or arrange a ride home for the patient.

Guidelines and Recommended Practices

Guidelines are "systematically developed recommendations that assist the practitioner and patient in making decisions about health care."[6] Recommended practices represent the association's official position on technical and professional practice. Guidelines and recommended practices are advisory and intended to guide practice while allowing for deviation when necessary.[8] During legal proceedings, however, guidelines, position

---

Box 3
Presedation history and physical evaluation by a registered nurse

General health

Height and weight

Obesity or recent weight loss

Current infection

Current medications (prescription or over-the-counter)

Current herbal use

Last food intake (fasting history)

Physical handicaps and level of mobility

Baseline vital signs and temperature

History of tobacco or alcohol use

Pain assessment (chronic or acute)

Cardiovascular

History of cardiovascular disease

Recent cardiac surgery or myocardial infarction

Angina, aortic stenosis, congestive heart failure

Presence of a pacemaker or implantable cardioverter defibrillator

Respiratory

Smoking history

Chronic cough

History of lung surgery or emphysema

Shortness of breath

History of tuberculosis, pneumonia, asthma, or bronchitis

Baseline oximetry reading

Airway assessment

Mallampati assessment or other, such as having patient open mouth, stick out tongue, and flex neck

Craniofacial abnormalities

History of sleep apnea

Neurologic

General affect, including behavior, speech patterns, gait

Level of consciousness and orientation

History of seizures, headaches

Motor abilities

Preexisiting neurologic deficit

Musculoskeletal

Muscle strength, mobility, range of motion

Use of orthopedic devices or prostheses

History of arthritis, scoliosis, fractures

Integumentary

Color (cyanosis or jaundice)

Temperature and texture

Skin turgor

Integrity of skin

Piercings

Gastrointestinal

Chronic diarrhea or constipation

Predisposition to nausea and vomiting

Time of last oral intake

Previous surgery or procedures

Renal/hepatic

Kidney function (eg, end-stage renal disease for revision of arteriovenous fistula)

Liver disease, including cirrhosis, hepatitis, anemia

Endocrine

Diabetes (most common abnormality)

From Odom-Forren J, Watson D. Practical guide to moderate sedation/analgesia. 2nd edition. St. Louis (MO): Elsevier Mosby; 2005. p. 22–3; with permission.

---

statements, recommended practices from national organizations, and recommendations from pharmaceutical companies can be presented as expected and acceptable standard of care.

Guidelines can decrease the number of adverse events. Variation in sedation practices prompted TJC to expand its sedation standards in 2001. These standards were updated in conjunction with the ASA and reflect the ASA's guideline for management of sedation by nonanesthesiologists.[6] Pittetti and colleagues[47] examined the efforts of one institution to establish TJC's guidelines and how the guidelines impacted adverse events during sedation. Procedural sedation was then monitored over a 3-year period with 14,386 cases. Adverse events occurred in 7.6% of patients. The most common adverse event was hyoxemia, defined as an oxygen saturation level of 90% or lower for more than 1 minute. The incidence of adverse events decreased significantly over time during the study. Further research is needed to evaluate whether a standardized approach to sedation will reliably decrease adverse events.[47]

SUMMARY

Serious adverse events with permanent sequelae or death are rare during nurse-monitored sedation;

however, to reduce the risk for sedation-related complications that lead to adverse events, practitioners should

1. Perform and document a thorough presedation evaluation including a history and physical examination.[5,6,8,48]
2. Use appropriate patient selection by assigning an ASA score to determine those who need further work-up.[6,8,48]
3. Obtain training in basic and advanced cardiac life support.[5,6,8,48]
4. Follow organizational guidelines, policies, and protocols.[8,48]
5. Know the pharmacology of the sedative and reversal agents.[5,6,8,29,37–39,48]
6. Titrate sedative dosing in each patient to the desired effect.[5,6,8,29,37–39]
7. Obtain and maintain continuous intravenous access, which is an emergency lifeline.[5,6,8]
8. Assess the level of sedation, vital signs, and oxygen saturation periodically and document every 5 minutes during the procedure.[5,6,8,29,37–39]
9. Use oxygen supplementation on all patients[5] or consider its use with moderate sedation and require its use with deep sedation.[6,8,29,37–39]
10. Use ECG monitoring in all patients[8,37,38] or, at a minimum, in all patients who have known cardiovascular disease.[5,6,29,39]
11. Consider capnography for patients who are undergoing deep sedation or prolonged procedures.[5,6,8,29,38,39]
12. Turn on alarms and keep them on.[6,8,48]
13. Use standardized discharge criteria to determine readiness for discharge.[5,6,8,29,37–39]
14. Follow guidelines to enhance patient safety.[6,8,29,37–39]
15. Explore learning opportunities to maintain competencies and keep patients safe.[5,6,8,29,37–39]

Future areas of research in clinical studies include safety and efficacy studies (eg, new agents, postdischarge adverse events, and definition of successful sedation); applications of new technology; and procedural sedation and analgesia adjuncts.[16] Research efforts must continue to determine the diagnosis of scenarios that can lead to adverse events.[42] No consensus exists on optimal dosing strategies, target depth of sedation, or definition of complications.[16] Large multicenter trials are needed that have standardized sedation protocols, standardized adverse event reporting, and standardized outcome measures. These trials have the potential to establish the true complication rate for each sedation level,

drug, and procedure to determine the best way to manage the patient and provide optimal patient safety.[16] In the meantime, perioperative nurses would do well to follow multidisciplinary guidelines that are available and to ensure proper education and competency to respond quickly to adverse events. The facility should support a sedation system that has prewritten scenarios of response with practiced personnel.

REFERENCES

1. Kohn LT, Corrigan JM, Donaldson MS, editors. To err is human: building a safer health system. A report of the committee on quality of health care in America. Institute of Medicine. Washington, DC: National Academy Press; 2000.
2. Donaldson MS. An overview of To Err Is Human: reemphasizing the message of patient safety. In: Hughes RG, editor. Patient safety and quality: an evidence-based handbook for nurses volume 1. Agency for Healthcare Research and Quality. Rockville (MD): US Department of Health and Human Services; 2008. AHRQ Publication No. 08-0043, 1-37-1-45.
3. Meltzer B. RNs pushing propofol. Outpatient Surgery 2003;4(7):24–37.
4. Odom-Forren J. The evolution of nurse monitored sedation. J Perianesth Nurs 2005;20:385–98.
5. Vargo JJ. Minimizing complications: sedation and monitoring. Gastrointest Endosc Clin N Am 2007; 17:11–28.
6. Gross JB, Bailey PL, Caplan RA, et al. American Society of Anesthesiologists task force on sedation and analgesia by non-anesthesiologists: ASA practice guidelines for sedation and analgesia by non-anesthesiologists. Anesthesiology 2002;96:1004–17.
7. Blike GT, Cravero JP. Pride, prejudice, and pediatric sedation: a multispecialty evaluation of the state of the art. Report from a Dartmouth Summit on Pediatric Sedation 2000. Available at: www.npsf.org. Accessed June, 2008.
8. Odom-Forren J, Watson D. Practical guide to moderate sedation/analgesia. 2nd edition. St. Louis (MO): Elsevier Mosby; 2005.
9. The Joint Commission. Hospital accreditation standards. Oakbrook Terrace (IL): TJC; 2008.
10. Cote CJ, Notterman DA, Karl HW, et al. Adverse events and risk factors in pediatrics: a critical incident analysis of contributing factors. Pediatrics 2000;105:805–14.
11. Cravero JP, Blike GT, Beach M, et al. Incidence and nature of adverse events during pediatric sedation/anesthesia for procedures outside the operating room: report from the pediatric sedation research consortium. Pediatrics 2006;118:1087–96.

12. Hertzog JH, Havidich JE. Non-anesthesiologist-provided pediatric procedural sedation: an update. Curr Opin Anaesthesiol 2007;20:365–72.

13. Fanning RM. Monitoring during sedation given by non-anaesthetic doctors. Anaesthesia 2008;63:370–4.

14. Sieg A, Hachmoeller-Eisenbach U, Eisenbach T. Prospective evaluation of complications in outpatient GI endoscopy: a survey among German gastroenterologists. Gastrointest Endosc 2001;53:620–7.

15. Bhananker SM, Posner KL, Cheney FW, et al. Injury and liability associated with monitored anesthesia care: a closed claims analysis. Anesthesiology 2006;104:228–34.

16. Miner JR, Krauss B. Procedural sedation and analgesia research: state of the art. Acad Emerg Med 2007;14:170–8.

17. Hooper VD. Management of complications. In: Odom-Forren J, Watson D, editors. Practical guide to moderate sedation/analgesia. St. Louis (MO): Elsevier Mosby; 2005. p. 82–106.

18. American Society of Anesthesiologists. Practice guidelines for management of the difficult airway. Available at: www.asahq.org/publicationsAndServices/Difficult%20Airway.pdf. Accessed August 13, 2008.

19. Patterson P. Should RNs be giving propofol in GI lab? OR Manager 2004;20:24–30.

20. Kremer MJ. Pharmacology. In: Odom-Forren J, Watson D, editors. Practical guide to moderate sedation/analgesia. 2nd edition. St. Louis (MO): Elsevier Mosby; 2005. p. 53–81.

21. Institute for Safe Medication Practices. Propofol sedation: who should administer? Available at: www.ismp.org/Newsletters/acutecare/articles/20051103.asp?ptr=y. Accessed August 13, 2008.

22. Zed PJ, Abu-Laban RB, Chan WWY, et al. Efficacy, safety and patient satisfaction of propofol for procedural sedation and analgesia in the emergency department: a prospective study. CJEM 2007;9:421–7.

23. Rex DK, Overley C, Kinser K, et al. Safety of propofol administered by registered nurses with gastroenterologist supervision in 2000 endoscopic case. Am J Gastroenterol 2002;97:1159–63.

24. Walker JA, McIntyre RD, Schieinitz PF, et al. Nurse administered propofol sedation without anesthesia specialists in 9152 endoscopic cases in an ambulatory surgery center. Am J Gastroenterol 2003;98:1744–50.

25. Heuss LT, Schnieper P, Drewe J, et al. Risk stratification and safe administration of propofol by registered nurses supervised by the gastroenterologist: a prospective observational study of more than 2000 cases. Gastrointest Endosc 2003;57:664–71.

26. Overley CA, Rex DK. A nursing perspective on sedation and nurse-administered propofol for endoscopy. Gastrointest Endosc Clin N Am 2004;14:325–33.

27. Rex DK, Heuss LT, Walker JA, et al. Trained registered nurses/endoscopy teams can administer propofol safely for endoscopy. Gastroenterology 2005;129:1384–91.

28. Philip BK. Sedation with propofol: a new ASA statement. ASA Newsl 2005;69(2). Available at: www.asahq.org/Newsletters/2005/02-05/whatsNew02-05.html. Accessed July, 2008.

29. American Society for Gastrointestinal Endoscopy. Sedation and anesthesia in GI endoscopy. Gastrointest Endosc 2008;68:205–16.

30. Rex DK. Review article: moderate sedation for endoscopy: sedation regimens for non-anaesthesiologists. Aliment Pharmacol Ther 2006;24:163–71.

31. VanNatta ME, Rex DK. Propofol alone titrated to deep sedation versus propofol in combination with opioids and/or benzodiazepines and titrated to moderate sedation for colonoscopy. Am J Gastroenterol 2006;101:2209–17.

32. Mandel JE, Tanner JW, Lichtenstein GR, et al. A randomized, controlled, double-blind trial of patient-controlled sedation with propofol/reminfentanil versus midazolam/fentanyl for colonoscopy. Anesthesia and Analgesia 2008;106:434–9.

33. Pambianco DJ, Jcrorie J, Martin J, et al. Feasibility assessment of computer assisted personalized sedation: a sedation delivery system to administer propofol for gastrointestinal endoscopy. Gastrointest Endosc 2006;63:AB189.

34. Shavit I, Keidan I, Hoffmann Y, et al. Enhancing patient safety during pediatric sedation: the impact of simulation-based training of nonanesthesiolgists. Arch Pediatr Adolesc Med 2007;161:740–3.

35. Silber JH, Kennedy SK, Even-Shoshan O, et al. Anesthesiologist direction and patient outcomes. Anesthesiology 2000;93:152–63.

36. Hooper V. Competence in patient management. In: Odom-Forren J, Watson D, editors. Practical guide to moderate sedation/analgesia. 2nd edition. St. Louis (MO): Elsevier Mosby; 2005. p. 146–54.

37. Association of periOperative Registered Nurses. Recommended practices for managing the patient receiving moderate sedation/analgesia. AORN J 2002;75:642–52.

38. American Society of PeriAnesthesia Nurses. 2006–2008 standards of perianesthesia nursing practice. Cherry Hill (NJ): ASPAN; 2006.

39. Society of Gastrointestinal Nurses and Associates. Statement on the use of sedation and analgesia in the gastrointestinal endoscopy setting. Available at: www.agna.org/resources/Sedation-pos.html. Accessed May, 2008.

40. Zuccaro G, Radaelli F, Vargo J, et al. Routine use of supplemental oxygen prevents recognition of prolonged apnea during endoscopy. Gastrointest Endosc 2000;51:AB141.

41. Vargo JJ, Zuccaro G, Dumot JA, et al. Automated graphic assessment of respiratory activity is superior to pulse oximetry and visual assessment for

the detection of early respiratory depression during therapeutic upper endoscopy. Gastrointest Endosc 2002;55:826–31.

42. Soto RG, Fu ES, Fila H, et al. Capnography accurately detects apnea during monitored anesthesia care. Anesth Analg 2004;99:379–82.

43. Lightdale JR, Goldman DA, Feldman HA, et al. Microstream capnography improves patient monitoring during moderate sedation: a randomized, controlled trial. Pediatrics 2006;117:1170–8.

44. Mallampati SR, Gatt S, Gugino LD, et al. A clinical sign to predict difficult tracheal intubation: a prospective study. Can Anaesth Soc J 1985;32:429–34.

45. Donaldson M, Gizzarelli G, Chanpong B. Oral sedation: a primer on anxiolysis for the adult patient. Anesth Prog 2007;54:118–29.

46. Chung F, Assmann N. Car accidents after ambulatory surgery in patients without an escort. Anesth Analg 2008;106:817–20.

47. Pitetti R, Davis PJ, Redlinger R, et al. Effect on hospital-wide sedation practices after implementation of the 2001 JCAHO procedural sedation and analgesia guidelines. Arch Pediatr Adolesc Med 2006;160:211–6.

48. Shepard S, Lofsky AS. Patient safety tips: conscious sedation (moderate sedation) in the office. The Doctor's Company 2007. Available at: http://www.thedoctors.com/KnowledgeCenter/PatientSafety/articles/CON_ID_001630. Accessed September 2008.

49. Martin ML, Lennox PH. Sedation and analgesia in the interventional radiology department. J Vasc Interv Radiol 2003;14:1119–28.

Incidence of Deep Venous Thrombosis in the Surgical Patient Population and Prophylactic Measures to Reduce Occurrence

Jennifer S. Barnett, RN, MSN, ARNP[a],*,
Linda J. DeCarlo, RN, MSN, MBA, CNOR, RNFA, ARNP[a,b]

KEYWORDS
- Patient safety • Deep vein thrombosis
- Pulmonary embolism • Venous thromboembolism
- Surgical patient • DVT prophylaxis

An astounding 200,000 to 600,000 people in the United States develop deep venous thrombosis (DVT) and pulmonary embolism (PE) annually. As many as 60,000 to 200,000 individuals die of PE, which makes it more deadly in the United States than motor vehicle accidents, breast cancer, or AIDS. DVT has been called a silent epidemic; approximately half the time the condition causes no symptoms. All too frequently, people die of PE without ever knowing they had a DVT.[1]

Public awareness of DVT increased in America after seeing former Vice President Dan Quayle experience a DVT.[1] David Bloom, a 40-year-old NBC news correspondent who died while covering the war in Iraq, heightened awareness even further. David Bloom's sudden death after experiencing leg cramps with associated PE has been an impetus to increasing public awareness of DVT and PE.[2] Despite this growing awareness, approximately two thirds of Americans know nothing about DVT, and more than half of individuals who are aware of DVT are unaware of risk factors, pre-existing conditions, or signs and symptoms of DVT.[1]

More than 23 million surgeries are performed in the United States yearly,[3] and every surgical patient is at risk for developing DVT or PE. DVT and PE are jointly referred to as venous thromboembolism (VTE). Although all surgical patients are at risk for VTE, many remain at higher risk because extensive operative procedures are being performed on individuals with greater medical comorbidities and advancing age.[4] The type of procedure and patient risk factors determine the potential for postsurgical VTE development.[3] As many as half of DVTs associated with surgery start intraoperatively.[5] Most hospitalized patients who develop symptomatic VTE are diagnosed after discharge from the hospital. What follows is a costly diagnostic and treatment process with the possibility of readmission. Complications are related to anticoagulation and long-term morbidity or death.[6] Problems associated with VTE could be avoided by the use of simple, cost-effective measures. Nurses participating in a surgical patient's continuum of care are in a unique position to ensure patient safety by increasing the level of awareness of DVT among patients, physicians, and hospital staff. Aggressive steps in using existing recommendations for VTE prevention can decrease the chance of the deadly complication of PE.

[a] Cascade Vascular Associates, 1802 South Yakima, Suite 204, Tacoma, WA 98405, USA
[b] 6028-58th Street West, University Place, WA 98467, USA
* Corresponding author. 3 Wilson Drive, Puyallup, WA 98371.
E-mail address: jbarnettarnp@hotmail.com (J.S. Barnett).

Perioperative Nursing Clinics 3 (2008) 367–382
doi:10.1016/j.cpen.2008.08.007

This article reviews the background and the incidence of VTE in surgical patients by surgical specialty, prophylactic measures to reduce occurrence, and nursing implications for practice (**Box 1**).

PATHOPHYSIOLOGY

In 1856, Rudolph Ludwig Karl Virchow, a German pathologist, identified a triad of factors that lead to intravascular coagulation. The factors of stasis, vessel wall injury, and hypercoagulability are as pertinent today as they were 150 years ago when identifying the pathogenesis of DVT formation (**Figs. 1** and **2**).[7–9]

DVT occurs when a thrombus consisting of red blood cells, platelets, and leukocytes forms in a large vein. Areas of slow or disturbed blood flow are the most likely location for a thrombus to either partially or completely block circulation. Thrombi can form where a vessel wall injury occurs intraoperatively. Injury can occur from the use of a tourniquet, insertion of an indwelling catheter, or mobilization of vessels to create exposure. Coagulation can be enhanced or fibrinolysis may be impaired. The result is a hypercoagulable state. Hypercoagulability can be caused by deficiencies in factors that inhibit coagulation (antithrombin III, protein C, protein S).[10]

Secondary hypercoagulable states may result from endothelial activation by cytokines leading to a loss of the normal anticoagulant surface functions of the vessel wall. The vessel wall converts to proinflammatory thrombogenic functions. Vasoconstriction causes venous stasis. The resulting increase in blood viscosity is the precursor to thrombus formation.[10]

Thrombi may form at any point along the vein wall, but most originate in valve pockets. A thrombus may extend retrograde, further proximally, or expand to completely fill the vessel. Thrombosis is often asymptomatic and resolves spontaneously via the fibrinolytic system through the mechanisms of recanalization, organization, and lysis.

Resolution of the thrombosis can be partial or complete.[8]

Fifty percent of DVTs start intraoperatively, with approximately 50% of them resolving spontaneously within 72 hours. The risk of symptomatic VTE is highest 2 weeks after surgery and remains elevated for 2 to 3 months.[5] When the condition persists, it can develop into a DVT and lead to a life-threatening PE.

Risk factors for developing a DVT can be divided into two categories: acquired and inherited (**Box 2**). The combination of patient risk factors plus type of surgery determines risk for developing a DVT. The American College of Chest Physicians (ACCP) has compiled data from prospectively validated evidence-based research studies to define risk groups of low, moderate, high, and highest to recommend prophylaxis either by category of risk or by surgical specialty.[2] Cancer increases the risk of DVT. Intrinsically, tumor production can affect coagulation parameters. Extrinsic factors that contribute to the pathogenesis of thromboembolism are indwelling access catheters used for chemotherapeutic agents, the chemotherapeutic agents, and venous stasis occurring because of weakness and decreased ambulation. Pancreatic, lung, gastrointestinal tract, and breast cancers are associated with a higher risk of DVT.[8]

Nutescu[2] described a study using a computer-based VTE screening tool used for patients on admission to the hospital. An electronic alert is sent to a patient's physician notifying him or her of the patient's risk of VTE. The ideal system goes one step further. It not only would identify a patient's risk for VTE but also would specify the AACP-recommended prophylaxis based on risk factors and type of surgery scheduled. To be successful, a VTE risk assessment tool must be easy to understand and implement. A combination risk assessment tool/prophylaxis order sheet in a patient's medical record could be completed collaboratively by the nursing staff and the medical staff.

Box 1
Definitions

Deep venous thrombosis: Blood clot in a deep vein.

Pulmonary embolism: Blood clot or fragment of a blood clot breaks loose from the wall of a vein and migrates to the lung, where it blocks a pulmonary artery or one of its branches.

Venous thromboembolism: The manifestation of a DVT or PE.

Thrombus: A stationary blood clot adhered to a vessel wall.

Embolus: A thrombus that has separated from a vessel wall and is traveling in the bloodstream to another location.

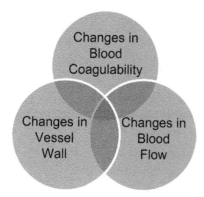

Fig. 1. Virchow's triad: relationship between coagulation factors.

of DVT risk, variation in the perception of risk factors, and concerns about the risk of bleeding with prophylaxis.[1,13] The most recent recommendations from the ACCP for antithrombotic and thrombolytic therapy were published in 2004 from the Seventh ACCP Conference.[6] The ACCP recommendations for VTE prophylaxis were developed using comprehensive literature searches of evidence-based research. The Seventh ACCP Conference on Antithrombotic and Thrombolytic Therapy guidelines have been used by the Joint Commission on Accreditation of Healthcare Organizations to create performance standards for VTE risk assessment and prophylaxis.[7,14] Prevention of VTE falls into two categories: mechanical and pharmacologic prophylaxis.

SIGNS AND SYMPTOMS OF DEEP VENOUS THROMBOSIS AND PULMONARY EMBOLISM

The clinical manifestations of DVT vary based on the size of the thrombus, the affected vein, and the adequacy of collateral circulation.[10] The classic symptoms of DVT include swelling, pain, and discoloration of the affected extremity.[11] Calf tenderness, low-grade fever, fatigue, tachycardia, and diaphoresis are also symptoms of DVT.[12] Physical examination may reveal a palpable cord of thrombosed vein, unilateral edema, warmth, or superficial venous dilation.[11] Because the clinical manifestations of DVT are so variable, objective testing and a thorough history and physical examination should be obtained.[10] The cardinal signs and symptoms of PE are shortness of breath, pleuritic chest pain, and mental status changes.[12]

METHODS OF PROPHYLAXIS

Despite risk factors being identified, VTE prophylaxis is underused because of a lack of awareness

Mechanical Prophylaxis

Mechanical measures are simple to implement and do not increase the risk of bleeding. People who are at low risk for developing VTE or have contraindications for the use of pharmacologic measures are good candidates for mechanical prophylactic measures, including early ambulation, foot and ankle exercises, passive range of motion exercises, graduated compression stockings (GCSs), and intermittent pneumatic compression (IPC) devices.[15] All of these measures improve venous return and reduce venous stasis in leg veins during the immediate postoperative period, when patients have decreased mobility because of pain.[16]

The advantages of using GCS, IPC, and foot pumps are that they carry no risk of bleeding or drug interactions. The disadvantages are that they require virtually constant use, and compliance is difficult to assess. The evidence of efficacy is limited because of variations in equipment

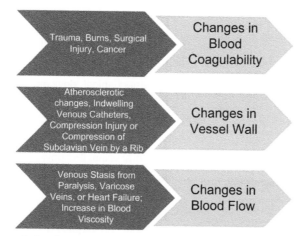

Fig. 2. Virchow's triad: coagulation factors.

Box 2
Deep Venous Thrombosis Risk Factors

Acquired risk factors

Female gender

Smoking

Age > 40 years

Obesity (body mass index > 29)

Hypertension

Malignancy/chemotherapy

Prior history of DVT

Prior major surgical procedure (within 3 months)

Trauma (especially pelvis, hip, or leg fracture)

Respiratory failure

General versus neuraxial anesthesia

Anesthesia > 3.5 h

ASA > 3

Indwelling venous catheters/CVP/arterial line

Surgery

Tourniquet > 50 min

Total hip/knee replacement

Planned postoperative admission to ICU

Immobilization (within 30 days)

Acute infection (urinary, respiratory)

Paralysis/paraplegia

Venous stasis/varicose veins

Congestive heart failure

Myocardial infarction

Atrial fibrillation

Diabetes mellitus

Inflammatory bowel disease

Pregnancy (especially 3rd trimester)

Postpartum

Oral contraceptives

Hormone replacement therapy (highest risk during first year of treatment, 45–64 years old)

Long plane trips (> 5000 km) and automobile trips

Intravenous drug abuse

Nephrotic syndrome

Thrombocytopenia

Antiphospholipid antibody syndrome (lupus)

Polycythemia

Thrombophelia

Inherited risk factors

Ethnicity (white, African American)

Sickle cell trait

Factor V Leiden

Protein C deficiency

Protein S deficiency

Prothrombin gene defect

Dysfibrinogenemia

Plasminogen disorders

Hyperhomocysteinemia

Elevated factor VIII

Elevated factor XI

Data from Refs.[1,7,8,14,17,25,28]

design, and they are often used in combination with pharmacologic treatment. Mechanical methods of thromboprophylaxis are safe and useful adjuncts to pharmacologic approaches.[17]

GCSs may reduce the risk of DVT by multiple mechanisms. Compressing the leg reduces the size of the veins and results in increased blood velocity, thereby reducing stasis. Reducing the size of the veins also improves the function of the venous valves and decreases pooling. GCSs provide greater compression at the ankle and augment the effect of the calf muscle pump. All of these mechanisms cause a reduction in venous pooling that can result in an alteration in the levels of clotting factors, which may lead to thrombus formation.[18]

Proper fit is necessary to prevent a tourniquet effect from GCSs that are too tight. They should be removed once a shift for 30 minutes to assess underlying skin.[15] Contraindications for using GCSs are certain dermatologic diseases, peripheral arterial disease, and diabetic neuropathy. Compression stockings have the potential to cause ischemic necrosis of the legs in patients with peripheral arterial disease.[18]

IPC devices simulate the effects of walking and weight bearing. Several studies have shown that mechanical devices (continuous-passive movement and IPC devices) increase the velocity of blood flow, reduce venous stasis, and reduce the incidence of DVT.[16] In addition to the mechanical process of increasing blood flow through the femoral veins, IPC devices have an antithrombotic effect on the components in the coagulation cascade.[19]

Devices vary by site of application, rate of inflation/deflation, pressure amplitude, and chamber inflation sequence.[19] Successful use depends on proper sizing and application of the sleeve containing the air chambers. Calf devices inflate and deflate to mimic the calf muscle pump.[9] The effect is simulation of the calf muscle stretching rather than simulation of muscle contraction. Elongation of the muscles in dorsiflexion of the foot increases the flow of blood in the superficial femoral vein fourfold.[19]

Early calf IPC devices used low pressure and slow inflation of a single air bladder. Current devices have multiple air chambers that produce graduated, sequential, and rapid inflation. The newer technology has been shown to improve hemodynamic response compared with the slower, low-pressure inflation of previous devices.[19]

Venous plexus foot pumps mimic the action of walking. The devices intermittently compress and relax the sole of the foot, which causes muscle contraction and improves venous blood flow.[9] Calf IPC has been proven to be superior to IPC of the foot.[19] Calf IPC or venous plexus foot pumps should not be used on patients with acute DVT, peripheral vascular ischemia, large, open wounds, skin grafts, or cancer of the extremity. If compression devices are not applied at the onset of bed rest or in surgery, an ultrasound should be performed to rule out DVT before initiating compression therapy.[20]

Intermittent compression devices are the safest and least invasive intervention used to decrease the incidence of DVT; however, their effectiveness is limited by poor compliance rates. To be effective, they must be used for the duration of bed rest—not just a few hours a day. The factors negatively affecting compliance include doctors, nurses, and patients not understanding the importance of IPC, no formal documentation system for the use of IPC devices, and nurses not noticing if an IPC device is ordered or if it is in good working condition.[15,21]

Common patient complaints about IPC include a feeling of warmth or having difficulty sleeping with the continuous inflation/deflation.[15] Patients most likely to fail IPC prophylaxis include persons who have cancer, persons with a past history of DVT, or individuals who are older than age 60. This higher risk group should be considered for more intensive prophylaxis.[22]

The most invasive mechanical prophylactic measure to prevent VTE is the placement of an inferior vena cava (IVC) filter. There are multiple indications for placement of an IVC filter. For example, patients who are not good candidates for chemical anticoagulation but need PE prevention may be considered for IVC placement. Preoperative placement of an IVC filter may be appropriate in patients with a history of DVT or PE who are about to undergo a lengthy neurosurgical procedure and have a risk of postoperative

bleeding.[4,23] Patients with a prior history of DVT who are undergoing a Roux-en-Y gastric bypass procedure for weight loss are also considered candidates for an IVC filter.[24]

Pharmacologic Prophylaxis

The clinical importance of administering anticoagulant therapy is to decrease the risk of long-term symptomatic VTE and prevent postthrombotic syndrome.[25] Anticoagulation therapy includes low-dose unfractionated heparin (LDUH), low-molecular-weight heparin (LMWH), synthetic pentasaccharides, warfarin, vitamin K antagonists, and aspirin.

Bleeding is the greatest concern when choosing anticoagulant therapy as a prophylactic measure to prevent VTE. Multiple studies have shown no increase in major bleeding with LDUH or LMWH, however. There is a slightly higher risk of minor bleeding with low-dose LDUH compared with LMWH.[13]

Heparin works as a catalyst, activating and binding to anti-thrombin III, an endogenous antagonist against several coagulation factors. The main effect of LDUH on the coagulation cascade is blocking thrombin and fibrin formation.[10,17] Dosing is based on weight and requires monitoring of partial thromboplastin time. Dose adjustments are made based on laboratory results. Low-dose unfractionated heparin can be administered intravenously or subcutaneously, depending on whether effects are needed immediately or within approximately 1 hour.[10,15]

LMWH activity is more focused than LDUH. The main effect of LMWH is inhibition of Xa, thus interfering with the coagulation cascade one step earlier than the action of LDUH.[17] The advantage of LMWHs is they do not bind to plasma proteins. The result is a more predictable anticoagulant dose.[10] Low-molecular-weight products are eliminated through the kidneys. Patients who have renal impairment, are obese, or are elderly should be considered at high risk for complication with the use of LMWH.[2] Patients with a higher risk for bleeding should be started on LMWH rather than LDUH.[15] Compared with LDUH, LMWH offers comparable or superior efficacy and a similar or lower risk of bleeding.[17] LMWH (eg, enoxaparin, dalteparin, tinzaparin, reviparin, and nadroparin) can be administered once or twice daily on an inpatient or outpatient basis without coagulation monitoring.[15] LMWH has a higher acquisition cost but is more cost-effective because it does not require partial thromboplastin time testing.[11,17]

There should be special consideration of patients receiving neuraxial anesthesia (eg, epidural and spinal anesthesia) with the use of LMWH or other heparinoids. These patients are at risk for the development of epidural or spinal hematoma, which can lead to paralysis.[26] Although the risk for serious complications is rare,[27] the risk is increased when a patient has an indwelling epidural catheter or receives concomitant use of nonsteroidal anti-inflammatory drugs, platelet inhibitors, or other forms of anticoagulation.[26] The risk of hematoma versus the benefit of regional anesthesia must be considered when considering appropriate patient care.[27] The 2003 Consensus Conference of the American Society of Regional Anesthesia[27] clearly indicated that regional anesthesia can be safely used with LMWH prophylaxis with careful attention paid to calibration of total daily dose and timing of the initiation and continuance of LMWH in relation to neuraxial anesthesia.

Fondaparinux is a synthetic pentasaccharide that binds to antithrombin III. It accelerates the action of antithrombin III to inhibit Xa.[2,17] Like LMWH, there is no need to monitor partial thromboplastin time. Fondaparinux should not be used in patients with renal impairment, and with fondaparinux there is a risk of hematoma with spinal anesthesia.[15,17] Unlike heparin, there is a concern that it cannot be reversed with protamine sulfate.

Fondaparinux has been shown to be more effective than LMWH for the first 7 to 10 days after joint replacement surgery. It is associated with an additional risk of bleeding if administered less than 6 hours postoperatively, however. If anticoagulant therapy is stopped after 7 to 10 days, an additional month of aspirin prophylaxis should be considered in high-risk patients. The effectiveness of fondaparinux is similar to warfarin, whereas aspirin is less effective.[25]

Warfarin is an oral anticoagulant with a different mechanism of action than LDUH, LMWH, or fondaparinux. Although heparin products block activated coagulation factors, warfarin alters hepatic synthesis of vitamin K–dependent coagulation factor precursors, which makes them resist activation.[17] The result is depletion of clotting factors II, VII, IX, and X. Dicumarol, another oral anticoagulant, is used less frequently because of erratic absorption and gastrointestinal side effects. Dosage regulation of warfarin and dicumarol is based on laboratory monitoring of prothrombin time and international normalized ratio (INR).[10]

Warfarin has the convenience of oral administration for inpatient and outpatient use. It also has a low acquisition cost. The narrow therapeutic range requires frequent monitoring, however. Its effectiveness is also affected by a large number of foods, antibiotics, and disease processes.[15]

There is also a long list of serious interactions with other drugs.[17] These influences make it difficult to regulate.[15] The slow onset of action and widely variable responses are disadvantages. It can take more than 3 days for the INR results to reach the recommended range of 2.0 to 3.0.[17]

No controlled studies have evaluated the effectiveness of warfarin as VTE prophylaxis. In the literature, there is discussion of warfarin being associated with less bleeding, yet information also indicates that warfarin may cause more bleeding than LMWH during extended prophylaxis. Evidence suggests that warfarin and LMWH have similar efficacy in preventing symptomatic VTE within 3 months of hip and knee replacement.[25]

Aspirin decreases platelet aggregation and is effective in prophylactic treatment of arterial thrombi. Venous thrombi are composed of fibrin and red blood cells, which is why aspirin is not considered an effective method of preventing VTE. The Seventh ACCP Conference on Antithrombotic and Thrombolytic Therapy advised that aspirin alone is not recommended as prophylaxis in any surgical patient.[15] More specifically, aspirin is not recommended for prevention of VTE after orthopedic surgery. It is less effective than LMWH or warfarin. Despite its ineffectiveness in preventing VTE, it is simple to administer, inexpensive, and safe. There is a risk of gastrointestinal bleeding, however.[25]

The decision about the best prophylactic therapy for a patient should be based on efficacy, safety, and cost.[2] The efficacy of treatment with GCS, IPC, LDUH, LMWH, warfarin, and aspirin varies significantly by patient populations. The value of reviewing the data from different trials is to provide insight to the overall problem of VTE and the importance of thromboprophylaxis in high-risk situations.[17]

ECONOMIC IMPLICATIONS

The price of VTE prevention includes the cost of mechanical devices, pharmacologic therapy, and diagnostic procedures. Although prevention may seem costly, it is much more cost-effective than delayed discharge or readmission because of VTE. It is impossible to quantify all of the economic issues involved, especially the cost of loss of life because of PE. The impact on a family cannot be assigned a dollar figure.[28]

A dollar figure can be assigned to the debilitating effects of venous postthrombotic syndrome. The quality of a patient's life can be affected by chronic leg swelling, pain, leg ulcers, or amputation. The medical resources consumed as a result of these complications in addition to the ongoing costs to the patient in the form of lost income are limitless.[11]

INCIDENCE AND PROPHYLAXIS OF VENOUS THROMBOEMBOLISM IN SURGERY

Two approaches to VTE prophylaxis are an individual patient risk assessment model versus a model based on surgical specialties. The risk assessment model ascribes prophylaxis by considering patient-specific risk factors and provides recommendations based on risk factor stratification. The most important drawback to the risk assessment approach is that this model has not been validated adequately. It is difficult to determine exactly where an individual patient lies within the continuum of thromboembolic risk factors to assign effective prophylactic care. As a result, this method becomes logistically complex and may lead to substandard treatment.[6] Prophylaxis based on a risk assessment model is seen in Appendix 1.

The second method used to implement VTE prophylaxis categorizes patients based on the surgical specialty providing care for the patient's primary disorder. The ACCP supports the model based on surgical specialties for determining VTE prophylaxis. Assigning patients to appropriate surgical groups is straightforward, and interventions are recommended using evidence-based guidelines.[6] Throughout the remainder of this section, please refer to Appendix 2 for a synopsis of guidelines according to surgical specialty.

Orthopedic Surgery

Patients undergoing orthopedic surgeries are at particularly high risk for developing DVT and PE.[3,4,7,29] The Agency for Healthcare Research and Quality[3] affirms that when prophylaxis is not used, more than 50% of patients undergoing major orthopedic surgeries experience DVT and up to 30% develop PE postoperatively. Even when appropriate preventive treatment is initiated, VTE is still clinically evident in almost 3% of orthopedic surgery patients. Hospital readmission after hip replacement is most frequently because of VTE.[4] A significant factor associated with the high incidence of VTE in orthopedic surgery is the nature of the surgery, which often renders orthopedic surgical patients immobile.[7] Another concern is the evidence that the use of tourniquets for more than 50 minutes leads to a greater incidence of DVT.[11]

Total hip replacement

Approximately 1 in 1000 people undergo elective total hip replacement (THR) yearly. Forty-two percent to 57% of THR patients who do not receive DVT prophylaxis develop DVT detectable by venography, and 0.9% to 28% develop PE. Fatal PE develops in 0.1% to 2% of these patients.[6]

Mechanical methods of VTE prevention used in patients undergoing THR, such as GCS and IPC, do reduce DVT but are not as effective as anticoagulant-based regimens. There is strong evidence against the use of aspirin, dextran, LDUH, GCS, IPC, or venous foot pump as the sole methods of VTE prophylaxis in hip replacement patients.[6]

Total knee replacement

There is a higher overall risk of DVT with total knee replacement compared with THR. Literature suggests between 41% and 85% of total knee replacement patients without prophylaxis develop postoperative DVT.[3,4,6,7,17] Fatal PE occurs in 0.1% to 1.7% of total knee replacement patients.[6] Recommendations for prophylactic treatment for total knee replacement are similar to those for THR. LMWH is favored over warfarin, but there may be an increased incidence of postoperative bleeding with LMWH, particularly if started early in the postoperative period.[4,6] When IPC devices are used reliably, they are a beneficial alternative to anticoagulants when anticoagulation therapy is contraindicated.[6]

Hip fracture repair

Advanced age and delayed surgery are two factors that place individuals undergoing hip fracture repair at particular risk for VTE.[6] Rates of DVT after hip fracture without prophylaxis are approximately 50%. Rates of fatal PE occurring 3 months after hip fracture repair are between 1.4% and 7.5%.[4] Patients should receive DVT prophylaxis with LDUH or LMWH during the preoperative period if surgery is going to be delayed more than 24 hours.[4,6] Prophylaxis recommendations are similar to those for replacement surgery. The appropriate use of VTE prophylaxis seems to reduce the overall risk of DVT by approximately 60%.[4]

Lower extremity fracture repair

Information is scarce regarding the incidence and prevention of VTE after lower extremity fracture repair. Several studies have documented an incidence of DVT between 43% and 45% in patients who did not receive prophylaxis with tibial plateau fracture repairs, however. The closer the fracture is to the knee, the higher the risk for DVT. Uncertainty exists regarding the efficacy and cost-effectiveness of VTE prophylaxis in cases of isolated fracture repair in regards to clinically significant VTE. Until further information is available, clinicians should decide on a case-by-case basis regarding treatment. It is reasonable in cases of isolated lower extremity fracture that thromboprophylaxis not be used routinely.[6]

Elective spine surgery

The limited data available regarding incidence of VTE in patients undergoing elective spine surgery indicate overt DVT rates of 3.7% and PE of 2.2%. The following are risk factors for these patients: surgery on the cervical spine versus the lumbar spine, advanced age, anterior or combined anterior/posterior approach, malignancy, prolonged surgery, and reduced perioperative mobility.[6] Elective spinal surgery patients without additional risk factors need no other preventive care other than early, persistent mobilization. Patients with additional risks may benefit from LDUH or LMWH alone. Alternatively, mechanical devices may benefit. Patients with several risk factors benefit from LDUH or LMWH used in conjunction with mechanical devices.[6]

Joint arthroscopy

Knee arthroscopy is the most commonly performed orthopedic procedure in the US,[6] with more than 3 million are performed each year globally.[30] Without prophylaxis, studies support that VTE occurs in 2% to 18% of knee arthroscopy patients.[6] Compared to major orthopedic surgery, the risk is relatively low. A paucity of evidence regarding the usefulness of thromboprophylaxis in this population makes it necessary for treatment to be decided individually. Early ambulation, when suitable, should be encouraged with LMWH used on patients with higher-than-usual risk.[6]

General Surgery

Studies that estimate incidence of VTE in general surgery patients without the use of thromboprophylaxis are no longer performed. No current research provides accurate estimates of incidence in this patient group. Screening studies performed in the 1970s and 1980s reported an incidence of DVT and fatal PE ranging from 15% to 30% and 0.2% to 0.9%, respectively. It is possible that rapid postoperative mobilization, extensive use of thromboprophylaxis, and advanced perioperative care have reduced current incidence. On the other hand, the incidence could be higher than previously reported because surgical patients are older, often have multiple comorbidities, and undergo more extensive procedures. The trend toward shorter hospital stays results in insufficient length of time for recommended VTE prophylaxis. Low-dose unfractionated heparin and LMWH have been found to reduce the incidence of VTE by at least 60% in general surgical patients and are recommended as routine thromboprophylaxis. Effective measures to reduce DVT and PE are LDUH and LMWH. Patients at high risk for bleeding should use mechanical prophylactic measures.[6]

Laparoscopic surgical interventions have been used more widely over the past several decades. There is a slight association between laparoscopic cholecystectomy and the activation of the coagulation cascade in addition to the stimulation of fibrinolysis.[6] Pneumoperitoneum and reverse Trendelenburg position generate venous stasis in the lower legs by reducing venous return. Generally speaking, however, incidence of DVT after laparoscopy is generally small at 1.4%. The Seventh ACCP Conference on Antithrombotic and Thrombolytic Therapy[6] claimed that there simply is not enough evidence to recommend the routine use of thromboprophylaxis in laparoscopic patients. If a particular patient is deemed to be at high risk, a brief prophylaxis with a current prophylactic routine could be considered.[6]

Vascular Surgery

The occurrence of VTE in vascular surgical patients is difficult to assess because during vascular surgery patients routinely receive perioperative antithrombotic agents (eg, aspirin or clopidogrel) and heparin or dextran intraoperatively. Vascular surgery patients remain at high risk for VTE because of advanced age, limb ischemia, extended surgical time, and possible venous trauma. Atherosclerosis may be considered an independent risk factor for VTE. Clinically evident VTE occurs during hospitalization or within 3 months after surgery in 2.5% to 2.9% of vascular surgery patients. Patients who undergo open resection of an abdominal aortic aneurysm or aortofemoral bypass seem to have a higher incidence of DVT than patients who undergo leg bypass surgery. The incidence of DVT for patients undergoing aortoiliac or aortofemoral surgery without prophylaxis is comparable to other types of abdominal and pelvic surgeries (approximately 21%). Endovascular repair of abdominal aortic aneurysm also has risks. One study showed a 6% postoperative incidence of DVT by ultrasound in 50 patients who underwent endovascular repair of abdominal aortic aneurysm.[6]

A study performed by VanRij and colleagues in 2004[31] showed that patients undergoing varicose vein surgery had a DVT incidence of 5% despite the use of thromboprophylaxis. Surgical management in this study included general anesthesia for saphenofemoral junction flush ligation, long saphenous vein stripping, and phlebectomies. There is a higher risk for DVT when patients undergo bilateral versus unilateral varicose vein surgery. Extended prophylaxis is recommended for varicose vein surgery patients who have multiple risk factors.[31]

The consensus is that patients without additional thromboembolic risk factors who undergo vascular surgery do not need routine use of prophylaxis.[6] Patients who undergo major vascular surgery with additional risk factors should begin prophylaxis with LDUH or LMWH after surgery, however.[6]

Neurologic Surgery

Neurosurgical patients have an approximate 22% risk of developing DVT.[3,4] Intracranial surgery carries a higher risk compared with spinal surgery. Length of surgery, surgery for malignancy, lower limb paralysis, and advanced age also increase the risk for VTE perioperatively and up to 15 months after surgery.[3,6] It is necessary for this patient group to receive some form of VTE prophylaxis. Mechanical prophylaxis is used commonly in neurosurgical patients because of the concern for intracrancial or spinal hemorrhage. Craniotomy patients have a reduction in DVT by 82% when given LDUH; however, pharmacologic prophylaxis should be used with caution in these patients. Studies show that the rate of postoperative intracranial hemorrhage is 2.1% in patients receiving postoperative LMWH compared with 1.1% in patients with mechanical or no prophylaxis. Current recommended treatment options include a combination of mechanical devices (IPC and GCS) or LDUH or postoperative LMWH. High-risk neurosurgery patients should have a combination of mechanical and pharmacologic prophylaxis.[6]

Gynecologic Surgery

Rates for VTE are similar for patients undergoing major gynecologic surgery compared with those undergoing general surgical procedures.[6] Advanced age, malignancy, previous VTE, prior pelvic radiation, and an abdominal approach are risk factors for gynecologic surgery patients. Early and persistent ambulation is recommended for those undergoing brief (<30 min) procedures.[6] There is uncertainty regarding risk of VTE after laparoscopic gynecology surgery. The decision regarding prophylaxis should be made using the individual patient risk assessment model.

Urologic Surgery

Major urologic surgery carries a 1% to 5% risk for VTE. Fatal PE is the most common cause of postoperative death in these patients and occurs in less than 1 in 500 patients.[4,6] Multiple risk factors, such as advanced age, malignancy, and lithotomy surgical position, are factors in the development of VTE in urologic surgery patients. The risk for patients undergoing transurethral prostatectomy seems to be low, however. In these patients, early ambulation is the only recommendation. Patients undergoing more extensive open procedures (eg, radical prostatectomy, cystectomy, and nephrectomy) should have routine prophylaxis with LDUH or LMWH. Patients who are actively bleeding or are at high risk for bleeding should be started on IPC or GCS or both until bleeding risk is diminished.[6]

Recent advancements in robotics for prostate surgery require patients to be in lithotomy position for an extended period of time. The use of IPC and GCS in addition to pharmacologic prophylaxis is recommended.

Trauma Surgery

Major trauma patients have the highest risk of developing VTE. DVT risk exceeds 50%, and PE is the third leading cause of death for persons who survive past the first day.[3,6] An increased number of injuries correlates with an increased incidence of DVT.[32] Many of these trauma patients require surgical intervention, and appropriate perioperative thromboprophylaxis should be initiated. LMWH should be started as soon as considered safe. If pharmacologic treatment must be delayed, mechanical prophylaxis may be used as an alternative. Patients who have a delay in prophylaxis or suboptimal prophylaxis who are at high risk for VTE should be screened for DVT by Doppler ultrasound. IVC filters are not recommended as a primary method of prophylaxis. Treatment should be continued at least until discharge or after for individuals with major immobility issues.[6]

Plastic Surgery

Few publications report rates of VTE with plastic surgery.[17] The risk for DVT and PE in face lifts has been reported at approximately 0.39% and 0.16%, respectively.[17,33] Abdominoplasty patients seem to run a 1.1% risk of DVT and 0.8% risk of PE.[33] The practice advisory on liposuction advises that IPC and LMWH be used for "higher risk" plastic surgery patients.[17] Unfortunately, further specific guidelines do not exist for thromboprophylaxis in plastic surgery patients.[17] Until more studies provide evidence-based guidelines, intervention must be considered on a case-by-case basis and take into consideration individual patient risk factors.

NURSING IMPLICATIONS

Regardless of the knowledge of the incidence of VTE and the effectiveness of VTE prophylaxis, appropriate preventive measures are frequently underused. A survey taken by surgeons revealed that up to 14% of patients undergoing general surgery, 12% of patients undergoing hip fracture repair, and 3% to 5% of THR and total knee replacement patients do not receive VTE prophylaxis.[3] According to the Association for periOperative Registered Nurses, "The safety of patients undergoing operative or other invasive procedures is a primary responsibility of the perioperative registered nurse."[34] VTE prophylaxis of perioperative patients is an area of opportunity for nurses to make a significant impact on patient safety.

Knowledge is the key to identifying patients at risk for VTE. Venous thromboembolism can be prevented by risk stratification, identifying appropriate measures, and knowing when and how to apply the appropriate measures in a timely manner. Risk stratification begins when nurses perform an in-depth history preoperatively and should be ongoing throughout the patient's hospital stay, particularly if conditions change. Once individual patient risk factors and surgical specialty have been identified, nurses have the responsibility to advocate for appropriate prophylaxis.[11]

Nurses have the responsibility to educate patients and family about VTE. Educating patients about why they are at risk and why specific prevention measures are chosen improves compliance and acceptance of treatment.[18] Education should start with basic postoperative teaching topics, such as the importance of leg exercises, early ambulation postoperatively, maintenance of hydration, avoidance of prolonged periods of inactivity, and avoidance of constrictive clothing. Frequent turning, coughing, and deep breathing along with

not raising the knee-gatch on the bed to avoid popliteal pressure must be emphasized.[10] Patients need to be reminded to avoid standing or sitting for extended periods of time and sitting with knees bent or crossed for long periods.[22] An explanation of how elevating legs when sitting promotes venous return and prevents venous pooling may create a lasting picture in a patient's mind.[10]

If elastic stockings or IPC device is ordered, an explanation of how the calf muscle pump works may reinforce the importance of compliance with these measures. Signs posted on the wall at the foot of the bed in patient rooms have been used in an attempt to increase compliance.[23] A similar sign could be used for patients with IPC devices. The signs can serve as a reminder to patients and nursing staff (**Fig. 3**).

When anticoagulant therapy is prescribed, patients need to understand the importance of postdischarge follow-up. Specifically, arrangements should be made so patients are clear about where and when to go for follow-up once they leave the hospital. It is important to stress the need to continue the medication after discharge, the laboratory monitoring required, and the risk factors for bleeding.[9,11,22] Patients need to be alert to signs of bleeding and know to notify their care provider if they experience unusual bruising, nose or gum bleeding, blood in the urine or stool, vomiting blood, abdominal pain, joint pain or swelling, back pain, headaches, or a change in level of consciousness.[9,10,22,35]

Nurses need to discuss prevention of bleeding while on anticoagulant therapy. Patients should be reminded not to use salicylates, ibuprofen, or other over-the-counter products that affect coagulation without consulting their physician. They should use a soft toothbrush and an electric shaver rather than a razor. Contact sports should be avoided, and nightlights should be used to prevent falls. A medic alert bracelet stating the medication being taken should be worn to alert emergency medical personnel. Patients also

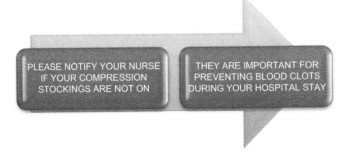

Fig. 3. Patient cues for DVT prophylaxis.

need to remind other health care providers that they are on anticoagulant therapy.[35]

Patients taking warfarin should be provided with a list of foods and medications that can alter their INR. They need to know the importance of following up with ordered laboratory tests to prevent excessive bleeding or blood clot formation.[9] Patients on warfarin need to know that tissue necrosis can occur from bruising at sites of fatty tissue such as the abdomen, breast, buttocks, and thighs.[22]

Teaching patients the signs and symptoms of DVT and PE is essential. They need to notify their health care provider immediately if there is redness, swelling, tenderness, pain, discoloration, or asymmetry of their legs or arms. They need to be instructed to call 911 if they experience unexplained shortness of breath, chest pain or palpitations, anxiety or sweating, or coughing up blood.

SUMMARY

VTE is an important patient safety concern. Nurses are in a key position to raise awareness of VTE prevention in the health care community and implement recommended prophylactic measures. Nurses can ensure that the most up-to-date recommendations are being used to prevent VTE in surgical patients by being involved in developing VTE prophylaxis guidelines in their facilities. Using the surgical specialty model as the primary method of determining VTE prophylaxis for surgical patients supports the recommendation of the Seventh ACCP Conference on Antithrombotic and Thrombolytic Therapy. The use of appropriate VTE prophylaxis prevents significant mortality, morbidity, and resource expenditures while ensuring patient safety.

ACKNOWLEDGMENTS

The authors would like to acknowledge Joanne E. Peterson, BEd, MAEd, in Guidance and Counseling, for her thoughtful critique of the manuscript, and Neal Van Der Voorn, MLS, MultiCare Health System Medical Librarian, for his assistance in researching multiple databases to provide an extensive source of references.

Appendix 1
Patient risk assessment model for venous thromboembolism prophylaxis

Risk Category	Risk Factors	VTE Incidence without Prophylaxis	Prevention Strategies
Low risk	< 40 years old undergoing minor, elective surgery No risk factors[a] General anesthesia < 30 min	Calf DVT: 2% proximal DVT: 0.4% Fatal PE: 0.1%	No specific prophylaxis other than early ambulation
Moderate Risk	< 40 years old undergoing major surgery < 40 years old undergoing nonmajor surgery with risk factors[a] 40–60 years old requiring general anesthesia > 30 min, without risk factors	Calf DVT: 10%–20% Proximal DVT: 2%–4% Fatal PE: 0.1–0.4%	LDUH (every 12 h), LMWH (≤ 3400 U/d), GCS, IPC
High Risk	> 40 years old undergoing major surgery 40–60 years old with risk factors[a] > 60 years old undergoing nonmajor surgery	Calf DVT: 20%–40% Proximal DVT: 4%–8% Fatal PE: 0.4–1.0%	LDUH (every 8 h), LMWH (> 3400 U/d), or IPC
Highest Risk	> 40 years old with multiple risk factors[a] > 60 years old undergoing major surgery Hip or knee arthroplasty, hip fracture surgery Major trauma, spinal cord injury	Calf DVT: 40%–80% Proximal DVT: 10%–20% Fatal PE: 0.2%–5%	LMWH (> 3400 U/d), fondaparinux, oral VKAs (INR 2-3), or IPC/GCS + LDUH/ LMWH

Adapted from Refs.[6,10,36,37]
[a] Risk factors include one or more of the following: advanced age, cancer, prior VTE, obesity, heart failure, paralysis, or presence of a molecular hypercoagulable state (eg, factor V Leiden, protein C deficiency) plus all of the items listed in **Box 2**.

Appendix 2
Surgical specialty model venousthromboembolism prophylaxis

Surgical Interventions	Recommended Prophylaxis	Prophylaxis Duration
Orthopedic THR	Usual high-risk dose LMWH 12 hbefore surgery or 12–24 h after surgery, or half the usual high-dose 4–6 hours after surgery then increase to usual high-risk dose on POD 1 OR Fondaparinux, 2.5 mg, started 6–8 hours after surgery OR Dose-adjusted warfarin started the eve before or the eve of the day of surgery (INR target 2.5, range 2.0–3.0)[6]	At least 10 days with a recommendation to extend up to 28–35 days[6]
Total knee replacement	Same as for THR Appropriate IPC use is a beneficial alternative to anticoagulation prophylaxis[6]	At least 10 days[6]
Hip fracture repair Contraindication secondary to high risk of bleeding Delayed surgery	Fondaparinux, LMWH at usual high dose, dose-adjusted warfarin or LDUH Appropriate IPC use is a beneficial alternative to anticoagulation prophylaxis Initiate LDUH or LMWH between admission and surgery[6]	At least 10 days with a recommendation to extend up to 28–35 days[6]
Isolated lower extremity fracture repair	No routine use of thromboprophylaxis[6]	N/A
Elective spine surgery No additional risk factors Patients with known malignancy, advanced age, neurologic deficit, previous VTE, or anterior approach Patients with multiple risk factors	Early, persistent mobilization Some form of prophylaxis (LDUH alone or postoperative LMWH alone); other options include periop GCS alone or with IPC) LDUH or LMWH with GCS and/or ICP	[a]

Knee arthroscopy		
Usual risk	No routine use of thromboprophylaxis other than early ambulation	[a]
For those at higher than usual risk for VTE following a prolonged or complex procedure	LMWH is recommended[6]	
General surgery		
Low risk (minor surgery, < 40 years old, no additional risk factors)	Early, aggressive mobilization	In selected high-risk general surgery patients, including those who undergo major cancer surgery, continue prophylaxis with LMWH after hospital discharge[6]
Moderate risk (minor surgery between 40–60 years old or have additional risk factors or major surgery but < 40 years old with no additional risk factors)	LDUH (5000 U every12 h), LMWH ($\leq$ 3400 U/d), GCS, or IPC	Until bleeding risk decreases, then follow previous guidelines[6]
Higher risk (nonmajor surgery, > 60 years old or have additional risk factors, or major surgery > 40 years old or have additional risk factors	LDUH (5000 U every 8 h) or LMWH (3400 U/d)	
High-risk (patients with multiple risk factors, > 40 years old, cancer, prior VTE)	LDUH (5000 U every 8 h) or LMWH (3400 U/d) + GCS and/or IPC	
High risk of bleeding	Mechanical prophylaxis (GCS or IPC)	
Selected high risk, including those who undergo major cancer surgery	Posthospital discharge with LMWH[6]	
Laparoscopic surgery	Aggressive, early ambulation (for patients with additional risk factors may consider LDUH, LMWH, IPC, or GCS)[6]	[a]
Vascular surgery		
Patients with no additional risk factors	No routine thromboprophylaxis	[a]
Major vascular surgery with additional risk factors	LDUH or LMWH usually started after surgery[6]	
Cancer surgery patients	As per specific surgery recommendation[6]	Continue 2–4 weeks after discharge[38]
Neurosurgery		
Intracranial	IPC $\pm$ GCS or LDUH or postoperative LMWH	[a]
High-risk patients	Combination mechanical and LDUH or LMWH[6]	

(continued on next page)

Appendix 2
(continued)

Surgical Interventions	Recommended Prophylaxis	Prophylaxis Duration
Gynecologic surgery Surgery ≤ 30 min, benign disease Laparoscopy with additional VTE risk factors	Early, persistent mobilization LDUH, LMWH, IPC, or GCS	Patients undergoing major procedures should continue prophylaxis until discharge[6]
Major surgery, benign disease, no additional risk factors	LDUH 5000 U twice daily or LMWH ≤ 3400 U/d or IPC started just before surgery continued until patient is ambulatory	Particularly high-risk patients (cancer surgery and > 60 y or previous VTE) continue prophylaxis for 2–4 weeks after discharge[6]
Extensive surgery for malignancy, and for those with additional VTE risk factors	LDUH 5000 U three times a day or higher dose LMWH (> 3400 U/d); alternative is IPC alone until discharged or combo of LDUH or LMWH plus GCS or IPC[6]	
Trauma No major contraindication and at least one risk factor for VTE	Start all trauma patients with LMWH as soon as safely possible	Continue until discharge from hospital, including inpatient rehabilitation[6]
If LMWH is delayed or contraindicated because of active or high risk for bleeding	IPC or GCS alone	Continue after discharge with LMWH or warfarin in patients with major impaired mobility[6]
Patients at high risk for VTE (spinal cord injury, lower extremity or pelvic fracture, major head injury, indwelling femoral venous line) who have not had optimal prophylaxis	Doppler ultrasound screening Recommend against the use of IVC filters as primary prophylaxis[6]	
Urology Transurethral or other low-risk procedures	Persistent, early ambulation	Optimal duration of treatment is uncertain; patients at high risk (elderly undergoing radical prostatectomy, hx of VTE, limited mobility) consider postdischarge thromboprophylaxis[6]
Major, open procedures	LDUH two to three times daily or IPC and/or GCS	
Patients at very high risk for or are actively bleeding	GCS and or IPC until bleeding risk decreases	
Multiple risk factors	Combination GCS and/or IPC with LDUH or LMWH[6]	
Plastic surgery	Intervention based on individual patient risk factors[34]	[a]

No specific guidelines regarding duration of therapy were provided in this surgical specialty by Seventh ACCP Conference on Antithrombotic and Thrombolytic Therapy.
[a] Guidelines serve as a reference point and are intended to be applied with clinical judgment by the prescribing provider. Individual patient circumstances should be taken into consideration when prescribing.

REFERENCES

1. American Public Health Association. Deep vein thrombosis: advancing awareness to protect patient lives. White Paper Public Health Leadership Conference on Deep-Vein Thrombosis 2003:1–12.
2. Nutescu EA. Assessing, preventing, and treating venous thrombo-embolism: evidence-based approaches. Am J Health Syst Pharm 2007; 64(Suppl 7):S5–13.
3. Agency for Healthcare Research and Quality. Prevention of venous thromboembolism. Available at: http://www.ncbi.nlm.nih.gov/books/bv.fcgi?rid=hstat1.section.61086. Accessed February 2, 2008.
4. Agnelli G. Prevention of venous thromboembolism in surgical patients. Circulation 2004;110(Suppl 5): IV4–12.
5. Kearon C. Duration of venous thromboembolism prophylaxis after surgery. Chest 2003;124:386S–92S.
6. Geerts WH, Pineo GF, Heit JA, et al. Prevention of venous thromboembolism: the seventh ACCP conference on antithrombotic and thrombolytic therapy. Chest 2004;126:338–400.
7. Summerfield D. Decreasing the incidence of deep vein thrombosis through the use of prophylaxis. AORN J 2006;84(4):642–5.
8. Kucher N, Tapson VF. Pulmonary embolism. In: Fuster V, Alexander RW, O'Rourke RA, editors. Hurst's the heart. 11th edition. New York: McGraw-Hill; 2004. p. 1593–615.
9. Crowther M, McCourt K. Get the edge on deep vein thrombosis. Nurs Manag 2004;35(1):21–30.
10. Woods SL, Froelicher ES, Metzer SA, editors. Cardiac nursing. 5th edition. Philadelphia: Lippincott, Williams & Wilkins; 2005. p. 239–41.
11. Chapman MW, Szabo RM, Marder RA, et al. Chapman's orthopaedic surgery. 3rd edition. Philadelphia: Lippincott Williams & Wilkins; 2000.
12. Kearon C. Natural history of venous thromboembolism. Circulation 2003;107(23 Suppl 1):I22–30.
13. Race TK, Collier PE. The hidden risks of deep vein thrombosis: the need for risk factor assessment. Crit Care Nurs Q 2007;30(3):245–54.
14. Ginzberg E, Banovac K, Epstein B, et al. Thromboprophylaxis in medical and surgical patients undergoing physical medicine and rehabilitation. Am J Phys Med Rehabil 2006;85(2):159–66.
15. Ramzi DW, Leeper KV. DVT and pulmonary embolism: part I. Diagnosis. Am Fam Physician 2004; 69(12):2829–36.
16. Brunicardi FC, Anderson DK, Billiar TR, editors. Schwartz's principles of surgery. 8th edition. New York: McGraw-Hill Companies; 2004. p. 1705.
17. Broughton G, Rios J, Brown S. Deep vein thrombosis prophylaxis practice and treatment strategies among plastic surgeons: survey results. Plast Reconstr Surg 2007;119(1):157–74.
18. Kehl-Pruett W. Deep vein thrombosis in hospital patients. Dimens Crit Care Nurs 2006;25(2):53–9.
19. Pearse EO, Caldwell BF, Lockwood RJ, et al. Early mobilization after conventional knee replacement may reduce the risk of postoperative venous thromboembolism. J Bone Joint Surg Br 2007;89(3): 316–22.
20. Mazzone C, Chiodo-Grandi F, Sandercock P, et al. Physical methods for preventing deep vein thrombosis in stroke [review]. Available at: http://www.thecochranelibrary.com. Accessed February 26, 2008.
21. Eisle R, Kinzl L, Koelsch T. Rapid inflation intermittent pneumatic compression for prevention of deep vein thrombosis. J Bone Joint Surg Am 2007;89(5): 1050–6.
22. Day MW. Recognizing and managing DVT. Nursing 2003;33(5):37–41.
23. Stewart D, Zalamea N, Waxman K, et al. A prospective study of nurse and patient education on compliance with sequential compression devices. Am Surg 2006;72(10):921–3.
24. Clarke-Pearson DL, Dodge RK, Synan I, et al. Thromboembolism prophylaxis: patients at high risk to fail intermittent pneumatic compression. Obstet Gynecol 2003;101(1):157–63.
25. Epstein N. Intermittent pneumatic stocking prophylaxis against deep vein thrombosis in anterior cervical spine surgery. Spine 2005;30(22):2538–43.
26. Prystowsky JB, Morasch MD, Eskandian MK, et al. Prospective analysis of the incidence of deep vein thrombosis in bariatric surgery patients. Surgery 2005;138(4):759–65.
27. BioPharm Communications, Llc. Venous thromboembolism: scope of the problem and the nurse's role in risk assessment and prevention. Clinical Impressions 2008.
28. Rowlings JC, Hanson PB. Neuraxial anesthesia and low-molecular-weight heparin prophylaxis in major orthopedic surgery in the wake of latest American Society of Regional Anesthesia guidelines. Anesth Analg 2005;100:1482–8.
29. Bjornara BT, Gudmundsen TE, Dahl OE. Frequency and timing of clinical venous thromboemolism after major joint surgery. J Bone Joint Surg Am 2006; 88-B:386–91.
30. Hoppener MR. Low incidence of deep vein thrombosis after knee arthroscopy without thromboprophylaxis: a prospective cohort study of 335 patients. Acta Oncol 2006;77(5):767–71.
31. VanRij AM, Chai J, Hill GB, et al. Incidence of deep vein thrombosis after varicose vein surgery. Br J Surg 2004;91:1582–5.
32. Stawicki SP, Grossman MD, Cipolla J, et al. Deep vein thrombosis and pulmonary embolism in trauma patients: an overstatement of the problem? Am Surg 2005;71(5):387–91.

33. Davison SP, Venturi ML, Attinger CE, et al. Prevention of venous thromboembolism in the plastic surgery patient. Plast Reconstr Surg 2004;114: 43e–51e.

34. Association of periOperative Registered Nurses. AORN position statement: statement on patient safety. Available at: http://www.aorn.org/PracticeResources/ AORNPositionStatements/Position_PatientSafety/. Accessed May 17, 2008.

35. Kaplan R. Deep vein thrombosis: prevention. An overview. CINAHL Nursing Guide. Available at: http:// search.ebscohost.com/login.aspx?direct=true&. Accessed February 26, 2008.

36. Bauer KA, Lip GYH. Overview of the causes of venous thrombosis: up to date online 15.3. Available at: www.uptodate.com/. Accessed February 26, 2008.

37. Pineo GF. Prevention of venous thromboembolic disease: up to date online 15.3. Available at: www. uptodate.com/. Accessed February 26, 2008.

38. Institute for clinical systems improvement. Health care guideline: venous thromboembolism prophylaxis. Available at: http://www.icsi.org/venous_ thromboembolism_prophylaxis/venous_thromboem bolism_prophylaxis_4.html. Accessed May 24, 2008.

Preventive Measures for Wrong Site, Wrong Person, and Wrong Procedure Error in the Perioperative Setting

Sharon A. McNamara, RN, MS, CNOR

KEYWORDS
- Wrong site surgery • Wrong side surgery
- Wrong patient surgery • Wrong procedure surgery
- Adverse events • Preventable adverse events

Newspaper headlines inform the public about the wrong leg amputated on a Florida man, a child has burr holes on the wrong side, and an adult with a subdural hematoma undergoes a craniotomy on the wrong side. These are some of the high profile cases that have the public questioning the safety of hospitals and have generated a flurry of activity in the United States health care system to put preventive measures into place to maintain quality, safe patient care. None of the professional practitioners participating in the procedures on these patients willfully performed these wrong site/side surgeries. In our current health care system, however, which is currently under development for a radical culture change, one of those practitioners could get the blame. The evolution in process is a change in philosophy of not pointing to the people but taking a broader view to look at the processes or systems in place to support those practitioners in doing the right thing every time. There have been recommendations and campaigns by professional associations on techniques to prevent wrong site surgeries, as discussed in the historical review. It was not until the Institute of Medicine opened the doors to the public and brought medical errors to the forefront that we came to a more serious consideration as to how to prevent wrong side/site, person, and procedure errors. This article reviews historically wrong site surgery prevention, scope of the problem, risk factors, prevention strategies, and performance measurement. Important aspects of zeroing in on safe perioperative processes, culture change, and involving the patient are examined.

HISTORICAL REVIEW OF PATIENT SAFETY AND WRONG SITE SURGERY PREVENTION

In 1994, the Canadian Orthopedic Association implemented "Operate Through Your Site," which was an educational program for surgeons targeted to reduce wrong site procedures (WSPs).[1] Leading the way in the United States, the American Academy of Orthopedic Surgeons (AAOS) Council on Education organized a task force in 1997 to research data on wrong site surgery. The task force's charge was to determine the prevalence of wrong site surgery and develop recommendations for preventing it. Data from the report demonstrated that from 1985 to 1995, 225 orthopedic wrong site surgery and 106 other surgical specialty insurance claims were filed. The cost of these wrong site surgeries averaged payouts of $48,087 to orthopedic patients and $76,167 to patients in other specialties.[2] Outcomes from this initiative resulted in an advisory statement on wrong site surgery, which stated: "The American Academy of Orthopedic Surgeons (AAOS) believes that a unified effort among surgeons, hospitals and other health care providers to initiate

WakeMed Health and Hospitals, 3000 New Bern Avenue, Raleigh, NC 27610, USA
E-mail address: smcnamara@wakemed.org

Perioperative Nursing Clinics 3 (2008) 383–393
doi:10.1016/j.cpen.2008.08.008
1556-7931/08/$ – see front matter

preoperative and other institutional regulations can effectively eliminate wrong-site surgery in the United States."[3]

The advisory statement spelled out effective methods for eliminating wrong site surgery. "Wrong-site surgery is preventable by having the surgeon, in consultation with the patient when possible, place his or her initials on the operative site using a permanent marking pen and then operating through or adjacent to his or her initials. Spinal surgery done on the wrong level can be prevented with an intraoperative X-ray that marks the exact vertebral level (site) of surgery. Similarly, institutional protocols should include these recommendations and involve operating room nurses and technicians, hospital room committees, anesthesiologists, residents and other preoperative allied health personnel."[3]

This advocates strongly for having the patient involved, marking the surgical site, involving the surgical team, and creating specific organizational policies to mandate the preventive measures. The AAOS did not stop there. They also advised that the surgical team should take a time out to confirm the patient's identity, ensure the correct procedure and site, check equipment, implants, and devices, conduct an additional check of the patient's medical record and radiologic studies, and addressing discrepancies before starting the procedure. This pause must include all members of the surgical team and leave time to ask questions if necessary. In 1998, the AAOS established the "Sign Your Site" campaign, which issued the advisory statement and created a logo, audiovisual programs, exhibits, and a mail campaign that delivered 20,000 informational flyers to orthopedic surgeons and operating room (OR) committees. The concepts for correct site surgery were also incorporated into the Academy's surgical skills courses, instructional courses, and specialty day meetings. Perhaps you have seen the marketing poster in the airport?

In 1998, the Joint Commission on Accreditation of Heath Care Associations (JCAHO) published Sentinel Event Alert Issue 6—Lessons Learned: Wrong Site Surgery. In that publication, factors were identified that may contribute to increased risk for wrong site surgery, which highlighted communication issues as the leading root cause. Three strategies for reducing the risk of wrong site surgery were suggested: marking of the operative site, oral verification of the site by the surgical team, and use of a safety checklist to include all aspects of verification.[4]

The 1999 Institute of Medicine report "To Err is Human: Building a Safer Health System" was published, and it dealt a serious blow to the US health care system. The purpose of the report was to promote safer processes in our health care systems and bring out into the open those serious concerns often hidden or discussed behind closed doors of the ORs and interventional units. Through its staggering numbers of reported patient deaths from preventable medical errors, this landmark publication heightened the awareness of patient safety issues for health care providers, patients, legislators, regulatory agencies, and the media. Media coverage quickly spread the word that the Institute of Medicine Report suggested that between 44,000 and 98,000 patients die in the United States every year as a result of medical errors. These numbers exceed the numbers of deaths attributed to motor vehicle accidents, breast cancer, and AIDS. The report also put a dollar value on the errors, stating that the national cost was estimated between $37.6 billion and $50 billion for adverse events and that between $17 billion and $29 billion were for preventable adverse events.[5]

One of the issues stated in the report is the lack of standardized nomenclature. The study used a definition for error from Gaba:[6] "An error is defined as a failure of a planned action to be completed as intended (ie, error of execution) or the use of a wrong plan to achieve an aim (ie, error of planning)." The definition of adverse event is "An adverse event is an injury caused by medical management rather than the underlying condition of the patient." An adverse event attributable to error is a "preventable adverse event."[7] The report is built around a four-tiered approach with recommendations to create health care environments that advocate for "establishing a national focus to create leadership, research, tools and protocols to enhance the knowledge base about safety; identifying and learning from errors through immediate and strong mandatory reporting efforts, as well as the encouragement of voluntary efforts, both with the aim of making sure the system continues to be made safe for patients; raising standards and expectations for improvements in safety through the actions of oversight organizations, group purchasers, and professional groups; and creating safety systems inside health care organizations through the implementation of safe practices at the delivery level. This level is the ultimate target of all recommendations."[5]

The North American Spine Society entered the safety campaign in 2001 through design of their SMaX Campaign, which encouraged surgeons to Sign, Mark, and X-ray surgical sites.[8] The radiography step is related to an additional safety check of a radiograph of the spinal level for site verification before beginning procedures on the vertebrae.

In 2001, a second report from the Institute of Medicine Committee on the Quality of Health Care in America was published. "Crossing the Quality Chasm: A New Health System for the 21st Century" focused on a call to action to redesign the health care delivery system. The movement is directed toward an efficient, cost-effective, quality, patient-centered, and patient-involved system that promotes an environment that supports patient and professional safety. The report advocated for new skills and new approaches with integration of information technology and alignment of payment policies that included addressing quality improvement and outcomes. Six aims for improvement will drive the needed changes in key dimensions of the current health system. These aims establish that health care should be

- *Safe* to avoid injuries to patients from the care that is intended to help them.
- *Effective* to provide services based on scientific knowledge to all who could benefit and refrain from providing services to those not likely to benefit (avoiding under use and overuse, respectively).
- *Patient-centered* to provide care that is respectful of and responsive to individual patient preferences, needs, and values and ensure that patient values guide all clinical decisions.
- *Timely* to reduce waits and sometimes harmful delays for individuals who receive and give care.
- *Efficient* to avoid waste, including waste of equipment, supplies, ideas, and energy.
- *Equitable* to provide care that does not vary in quality because of personal characteristics such as gender, ethnicity, geographic location, and socioeconomic status.[9]

In 2002, the National Quality Forum published a report, "Serious Reportable Events in Health care." The report identified 27 "never events," which are events that were considered preventable and should never have happened. Surgery performed on the wrong body part was on the list. Surgery on the wrong patient and performing the wrong procedure were listed with additional specifications and implementation guidance for each.

In 2003, the Joint Commission on Accreditation of Health Care Organizations (JCAHO) held a Wrong Site Surgery Summit. JCAHO collaborated with numerous professional associations: the American Hospital Association, American College of Surgeons, AAOS, Association of periOperative Registered Nurses, American Medical Association, and more than 20 other organizations. The goal of the summit was to achieve consensus on the adoption of a standard protocol for preventing wrong site, wrong procedure, and wrong person surgery. After soliciting input, specific recommendations and consensus on the principles of prevention, the Universal Protocol for preventing wrong site surgery was birthed.

In October 2003, AAOS produced "sign–your-site a checklist for safety" tool.[2]

On June 20, 2004, the Association of periOperative Registered Nurses (AORN) Patient Safety First Campaign spearheaded its inaugural National "Time Out" Day. The observance was endorsed by the American College of Surgeons, American Society of Anesthesiologists, American Society for Health Care Risk Management, and the American Hospital Association. The purpose of the day was to increase awareness of the Joint Commission's Universal Protocol for preventing wrong site, wrong procedure, wrong person Surgery. Concurrently, the AORN's Correct Site Surgery Tool Kit was rolled out to 40,000 members. An additional 50,000 copies of the tool kit were sent to chief executive officers and risk managers across the United States to emphasize the importance of standardizing the implementation of the Universal Protocol. The kit contained tools to assist with implementation: an educational CD-ROM, free independent study activity, a copy of the Universal Protocol and the frequently asked questions, a plasticized pocket reference guide for implementing the JCAHO Universal Protocol, and the JCAHO "Speak Up" safety initiative patient safety brochure. AORN continues to hold National Time Out days every year and provides free resources to reinforce the necessity to implement and monitor the Universal Protocol for prevention of WSPs and improved care for patients.[10]

In 2006, the Joint Commission International Center for Patient Safety developed the international patient safety goals. Six goals were created; fourth goal is elimination of wrong site, wrong patient, wrong procedure surgery. The goal includes the criteria for marking the site, conducting a time out, and using checklists. These requirements are mirrored to the Universal Protocols best practices.[11] In July 2007, the Council on Surgical and Perioperative Safety, a coalition of seven US organizations that represents the perioperative care team, endorsed as one of its core principles "that all measures will be used to ensure correct patient, correct site, correct procedure surgery, including implementation of the Universal Protocol of the Joint Commission is recommended and support of the Time-Out before surgery or initiation of an invasive procedure."[12] The coalition consists of the following member organizations: AORN, the American College of Surgeons, the American Society of Anesthesiologists, the American Association of Nurse Anesthetists, the Society of Peri-Anesthesia Nurses, the Association of Surgical Technologists, and the American Association of Surgical Physician Assistants. Convening this group of practitioners for the select goal of safety in surgical and interventional areas is groundbreaking; the collaborative work is expected to support consensus work among practitioners in our health care system to create, maintain, and monitor processes to prevent WSPs.

In June 2008, the World Health Organization (WHO) held the Second Global Patient Safety Challenge: Safe Surgery Saves Lives. The WHO surgical safety checklist was launched to provide surgical teams across the globe an international tool "to ensure that patients undergo the right operation at the correct body site, with safe anesthesia, established infection prevention measures and effective teamwork for safer care."[13]

STATEMENT OF THE PROBLEM AND IMPACT

The importance of a concerted effort to examine WSPs and their effects is substantiated by the fact that these occurrences are considered preventable adverse events. The National Quality Forum includes wrong site surgery events on its list of serious reportable events, which are frequently referred to as "never events." WSPs include wrong person, wrong side or site, wrong spinal level, wrong organ, wrong implant, and wrong nerve block. WSPs can occur in any area of the hospital or ambulatory setting and are not limited to surgical areas. The risks are also present in procedural areas, such as the cardiac catheterization laboratory or interventional radiology suite and during procedures performed on patient units, in ambulatory care facilities, or in a physician's office, where more complex procedures are performed routinely. Despite the ambitious efforts of many professional organizations, agencies, individual facilities, and practitioners to eliminate WSPs, the numbers have not declined. For example, the Joint Commission database recorded 88 cases in 2005, and the most current data (from March 31, 2007) recorded 552 wrong site surgeries. WSP is the most frequently reported category of sentinel events, and communication is the primary area of risk.[14]

In Pennsylvania, all hospitals and ambulatory surgical centers are mandated to report wrong site surgeries and near misses. From June 2004 through December 2006, 427 reports were filed,

253 near misses were reported, and 174 surgical interventions were started on the wrong patient, procedure, side, or part. Eighty-three patients' incorrect procedures were performed to completion.[15] This leaves questions as to whether reporting is improving as provision for secure, anonymous, and mandatory sites to facilitate reporting are provided, the punitive culture is changing, or the number of cases reported are actually increasing. Are these incidents still being underreported? As we move toward a culture of safety in which we examine processes in contrast to the old finger-pointing blame-and-shame game to punish individuals, we have the potential for continued improvement in practice and reporting. It is obvious, however, that we have not eliminated WSPs.

RISK FACTORS FOR WRONG SITE SURGERY

Inabilities to understand the full scope of the problem are not a reason for inaction, because many of these sentinel events are preventable. These happenings are detrimental to patients, practitioners, and organizations. Patients initially seem to be the only victims, with the possibility of emotional or permanent physical injury or death. Practitioners take an oath to do no harm, there is an altruistic facet to their choice of profession, and causing harm to a patient can be devastating to an individual when the error is actually related to process or culture, all of which create another victim. The organization risks loss of trust not only from patients, their family, and the community but also from the practitioners who depend on the culture in which the evaluation of the incident is completed. I contend that many people fall victim in potentially preventable adverse events.

Identification of risk factors for individual procedures can assist in developing preventive methods and herald particular circumstances or events that increase the potential for a WSP. The Joint Commission identified multiple factors in their reviews of WSPs: multiple surgeons involved in a procedure, multiple procedures being performed, time pressures, unusual patient characteristics, failure to involve a patient in identification of the correct site, poor communication among the perioperative team caring for the patient, and reliance solely on the surgeon for determining the correct site.[14] Other contributing factors that could lead to a WSP include two patients with the same name, emergency procedures, morbid obesity, and unusual patient anatomy.

The American College of Surgeons targeted key high-risk processes from actual risk cause analyses that related to WSPs. Communication breakdown among team members and with the patient and family ranked highest. Cultural factors, such as hierarchy and intimidation, were included. The patient preparation process demonstrated issues with incomplete patient assessments, including not checking medical records, radiographs, and other reports. The procedure for preparing the OR illuminated numerous issues, such as unavailable patient information, staffing levels and competency, resident supervision, lack of safety policies and protocols, and distractions, including various individuals' emotional and physical status and environmental influences. The surgical scheduling process was also mentioned.[16] When considering an electronic medical record system, the scheduler and the practitioners must be alert to inadequacies of the system that could support choosing the wrong patient or the wrong visit and thus transferring current information to the wrong patient's chart. Information that comes from an outside source in any form must have patient information validated.

In their research of the literature and numerous data bases to investigate prevalence of WSPs, Seiden and colleagues[17] discovered many of the previous findings. The categories they chose to use were human factors (eg, personnel changes, workload, environment, and lack of accountability), patient factors involving sedation and confusion of the patient about the procedure, and procedure-related aspects such as room change for a patient before surgery, patient position changes, wrong site being prepped or draped, and lack of cross checks. Incorrect specimen labeling has resulted in a procedure being performed on a wrong patient. Patient stickers for labeling specimens must be removed at the end of a procedure to ensure that the next patient's specimen is not labeled with the previous patient's information. Consequently, if pathology results indicate additional surgery, a patient may fall victim to a WSP.

A discussion on potential barriers to implementation of the Universal Protocol is important because these barriers increase the possibility of risk. My own experiences and discussions with other perioperative directors identified pushback as a first reaction from staff and surgeons. This lack of buy-in related to concern regarding the possibility of increasing the work load and decreasing efficiency. Surgeons were hesitant to move toward a standardized approach and "cookie cutter" medicine, and adaptation to the change in culture was slow. Some staff performed the time out robotically, and the team performed under an assumption of safety. We also discussed diverse staff competency, ranging from novice to expert nurses. This variance in competency and experience could create staff hesitancy to challenge a surgeon to do a time out or question a possible error. These types of behavior are found throughout the literature along with organizations seeming to put the cost or return on investment benefit before quality and safety benefits. Each of these carries a level of risk for enabling processes—or lack of—that leave room for error.

Two other important considerations for risk in performance of WSP are (1) the pressure to produce and (2) environmental noise and distractions. The constant pressure for efficiency and decreased turnaround time may influence practitioners in taking dangerous short cuts that increase the potential for error. The hectic pace at the start of a procedure can have part of the team moving forward without the proper safety checks (eg, the surgeon starting the incision before the "time out"). Current OR and interventional suites are frequently outfitted with music systems intended to provide a tranquil atmosphere, but depending on a surgeon's choice of music and the favored genre of the other professionals, this could be a major aggravation or distraction. In addition to music, there are various alarms that cannot be silenced, numerous pagers and telephones that may need answering, suction machines, and smoke evacuators, all demand the attention of the circulating nurse and accost the ears and senses of the team. These distractions take the attention away from the patient and the procedure at hand and leave room for error.

Certain specialties are rising to the top of the risk list in the literature. Orthopedic surgery seems to have a higher risk of WSP. The AAOS has a long history of advocating for prevention of WSP, which may impact increased reporting. Opportunities for lateralization errors and the higher volume of cases in orthopedics may relate to the increased risk and percentage of WSPs in orthopedics.[18] In their review of claims from twenty-two insurers, an AAOS task force found that orthopedic procedures accounted for 68% of WSPs.[19] The Joint Commission reported 41% of wrong site surgeries for orthopedics in 2001.[20] A survey of 1050 hand surgeons resulted in information that 21% admitted to one wrong site surgery and an additional 16% reported near misses. Most frequent locations were hand, wrist, and fingers.[21]

The number and variety of possible areas of risk demonstrate that potentially every patient may be exposed to a WSP. Would this information not validate for every practitioner the need for preventive measures in every surgical and interventional arena?

STRATEGIES TO PREVENT WRONG SITE PROCEDURES

Communication has been identified as the primary reason for medical errors by the Joint Commission. It seems fitting that many of the strategies that are discussed revolve around some form of communication. Transitions or handoffs of a patient's care are areas of high risk for communication breakdowns. Improving teamwork and continuity of care in relation to these transitions—whether from nurse to nurse, physician to nurse, or patient to doctor—is addressed in this article relative to WSP. See other articles in this issue for details on the specific strategies that can be used to prevent WSP.

Current tools and strategies being implemented across the world demonstrate increasing awareness of the issue of WSP, the need to come out of the climate of secrecy into a culture of acknowledgment of the error, learning from the investigation, developing creative methods for prevention, and sharing those finding so that no other patient has to suffer the same devastating events. Movement toward this culture change is not always fluid. Leadership is important in creating and maintaining the metamorphosis in culture to eradicate preventable WSPs. It is obvious from the historical review that many key professional associations stepped forward to lead the charge. Coming to consensus on criteria for the Universal Protocol was monumental. Administrative support from the individual health care institutions in policy setting, education, marketing, roll out, and measurement of the quality improvement efforts to prevent WSP is imperative to success. This support includes medical, surgical, interventional, nursing, and allied staff that are enlightened and can act as peer examples to lead the move to a culture of safety.

Robert Wachter, MD,[22] speaks to the fact that providing data is useful but telling error or near-miss stories is key to motivating practitioners to do things differently. Using analogies from other industries, such as the Aviation Safety Reporting System, National Aeronautics and Space Administration, Federal Aviation Administration, or Toyota, is not often convincing to physicians because they see health care as far more complex than flying an airplane or making an automobile. The system/process aspects of these high-reliability organizations may provide valuable insight to systems thinking, but selling them as the main campaign is difficult for physicians. Many physicians have never performed a WSP or had a near miss and find it incomprehensible that this would happen to them. Encouraging well-respected clinicians to share their story is compelling in creating understanding that a WSP can happen to even the most detailed physician.

The Universal Protocol made mandatory by the Joint Commission in 2004 seems to be the gold standard for processes to prevent WSP. The Universal Protocol grew out of a summit of medical and surgical professional organizations representing a large portion of the practitioners and organizations that have the potential of being affected by and have the ability to prevent a WSP. Consensus was reached by this group on the creation of the Universal Protocol, which would facilitate a specific standardized approach to preventing WSPs. The protocol contained many of the requirements found in the AAOS and North American Spine Society initiatives but with further emphasis on ensuring verification processes, marking the site, and taking a "time out" or final verification immediately before starting the procedure.[24] Kwaan and colleagues[23] analyzed data compiled from a large malpractice insurer between 1985 and 2004. More than 3 million surgical procedures were evaluated for wrong site surgeries. Twenty-five wrong site surgeries were found, not inclusive of spine surgeries. Ten of 13 charts reviewed demonstrated minor injury to patients, two procedures resulted in temporary major injuries, and one patient sustained permanent injury. An interesting conclusion by the authors, the Joint Commission's Universal Protocol may have prevented eight of these wrong site surgeries. The numbers in this example also demonstrate the difficulty in establishing rates for WSP.

Currently, the Joint Commission, Joint Commission International, and WHO[25] are collaborating on the issue of performance of correct procedure at correct body site. There is agreement that an organizational policy describing a standardized approach to ensure that correct procedures are consistently performed on correct patients needs to be in place in the organization. An informed consent process is in place that advises patients regarding all aspects of their care, including the proposed procedure, alternatives, and risks and benefits in a language that patients can understand. Three other areas of agreement needed are preprocedural verification, marking of the procedure site, and conducting a time out, all of which are aspects of the Universal Protocol.

As noted in the section on risks, the process for preventing WSPs should begin with the surgical scheduling of a patient's procedure. Important aspects to be considered for precision are the correct name of the patient, correct procedure with correct spelling, and, if laterality is involved, "left" or "right" side is spelled out. With the new electronic medical record systems, ensuring that this is the correct person and the correct visit is important. Other important information includes any special considerations for this patient, such as latex allergy, morbid obesity, or special implants that need to be ordered. The verification process of the correct person, procedure, and site should be a repetitive process (with patient involvement, if possible) that follows the patient through the entire continuum of care—upon admission to the facility, before the patient leaves the preoperative area to go to the procedure area or OR, and as care is transferred between caregivers. Once the patient is in the surgical or procedure room before beginning the procedure, relevant documentation is reviewed, labeled images are checked on the viewer correctly or pulled up electronically accurately, and special equipment and implants are immediately available.

The second requirement of the protocol mandates marking the operative site. The unambiguous, indelible mark should be placed at or near the incision site so it is visible after prepping and draping. The intent is to have the person who is performing the procedure mark the site, with the patient participating—awake and aware, if possible. The nonoperative site should not be marked, and the method of marking should be consistent across the enterprise. Single-organ cases do not require marking, but all cases that involve laterality, multiple structures (eg, fingers, toes, lesions), or multiple levels of the spine should be marked. It is expected that in addition to the external spine level mark, special intraoperative radiographic techniques should be used to mark the exact vertebral level. Concern regarding sterility of the mark has been unfounded.[26]

The third requirement states that a time out should be conducted immediately before starting the procedure. During this time out, which takes place in the location where the procedure is completed immediately before starting the procedure, the entire operative team is actively involved, and the correct patient, side, site, procedure, patient position, and proper implants and equipment are agreed on. If there is any discrepancy in the processes, there must be a policy and system to reconcile the differences.[24] The process needs to be documented, and checklists are one of the strategies recommended to confirm that a comprehensive, consistent, effective preoperative verification process was completed. Checklists also act as a good trigger for the practitioner to be sure all criteria are completed and negate the need to depend on memory systems, which can fail.

Examples of checklist are available in the literature and are frequently accompanied by discussions of implementation in addition to policies and other resources. An excellent article with numerous resources outlining implementation at the Children's Hospital in Boston could assist in development of policies, an education program, documentation suggestions, marketing, and measurement methods. This article has examples of the preoperative assessment and the time-out checklist criteria.[27] At the University of California, San Francisco Medical Center, Charlene Bennett, RN, MS, challenged her staff to come up with an acronym so the staff could remember the elements of the time out. The staff came up with a creative, catchy acronym: APPLE PIE (Antibiotics, Patient's name, Procedure, Laterality, Equipment, Position, Implants, Everyone participates). The slogan "The Items for a Time-Out Are as Easy as Apple Pie" made remembering the elements easy and patient safety fun and was more likely to energize compliance.[28] UMass Memorial Medical Center in Worcester, MA uses an electronic record that can create its own challenges for documenting the elements of a time-out verification. Their process involved using laminated cue cards to communicate the new process before implementing the one-page checklist that is completed by the circulating registered nurse. The electronic record contains all the elements and leaves no questions for the staff as to what needs to be agreed on and documented as part of the permanent patient record.[29] The AORN Tool Kit, which can be accessed and downloaded at www.aorn.org, provides another example of a checklist that includes sections for preoperative verification, marking the site, and time-out criteria. Checklists posted in the procedure room to act as memory joggers relieve reliance on memory systems that often fail in the organized chaos of the operating/procedure rooms.

Preliminary findings from the Pennsylvania Patient Safety Reporting System demonstrated that in 16 in-depth queries about near-miss events and six wrong site surgeries, all of the near-miss events involved a checklist for documentation of the verification process but only four of the six wrong site events involved a checklist. This finding is statistically significant per chi-square test and suggests that checklists have value in identifying risks in documentation variances that may lead to WSPs.[30]

An area that is problematic in complying with the Universal Protocol involves procedures completed on the patient units. Lankenau Hospital in Pennsylvania developed a system in which the time-out checklist is attached to the specific instrument trays that are used in procedures on the patient units. The central sterile processing department collaborated by placing the checklists and putting a bright green sticker with "time out" on the cart where the trays are stored. These cues serve to identify the tray for a procedure needing a "time out," and the document becomes the written verification of the process. Lankenau Hospital has seen a decrease in bedside events related to WSP.[31]

Several forcing mechanisms are being used to reinforce the implementation of a time out. The Methodist Hospital in Houston, TX developed a brightly colored reprocessable tent with the words "time out" printed boldly on it. This device is placed over the first instrument to be used in the procedure to stimulate team participation and compliance with the Universal Protocol time out. They have achieved a 95% compliance rate.[32] Several surgical supply companies have produced disposable scalpels with a cover that slides over the blade and handle with the words "time out." The function of having to remove the sleeve is meant to trigger the verification pause. Some OR staff keep the scalpel on the back table out of reach of the surgeon until the time out is completed.

The staff at Glenbrook Hospital in Illinois has found that scripting gives nurses who are not assertive communicators a tool they can rely on for consistency. They have developed a generic script that lays out the dialog to verify the six elements of the Universal Protocol. This script has decreased inconsistencies in the communication process and reduced the risk of errors in surgery.[33]

A strategy I would like to share is collaboration among hospitals in a geographic region to establish processes to meet the Universal Protocols elements as a community team. At three operative/invasive sites for WakeMed Health and Hospitals in Raleigh, NC, our surgeons also practiced at two other regional competitor hospitals, REX and Duke Raleigh. We frequently played the game of the surgeons telling us how they did not have to do these processes at the other hospitals. The directors of surgical services at the five hospitals came together and standardized the policies, procedures, and roll out dates for the various stages of the Universal Protocol. It worked like a charm, and we work closely to standardize as many practices as we can to facilitate safer, quality care for our community.

Technology has not taken a back seat to creating innovative methods to prevent WSPs. Richard A. Chole, MD, believed that a fail-safe marking system was needed. His invention involves a special wristband, marking pen, and CheckSite alarms. Once the site is marked, the special label on the pen is peeled off and placed on the wrist band. This label in place blocks a signal emitted by a chip in the wrist band that potentially activates as a patient proceeds into the OR through the threshold fitted with the alarms. If there is no label, the alarm, which can be set for a gentle sound or a visual clue, sounds to alert the staff of the risk.[34] Another hi-tech invention similar to the CheckSite system is a radio frequency identification technology that encodes patient information on a SurgiChip that can be electronically read by a handheld reader to verify correct information before surgery commences.[35] No matter what the process that is put into place, the importance of having all practitioners (the surgical team) actively involved, centered on the individual patient, and attending to that patient's needs ensures that a correct procedure cannot be overemphasized.

PERFORMANCE MEASUREMENT

As we move toward a culture of safety, an increasing awareness surfaces of the need to create proactive approaches to identify potential risks, put preventive measures into place, and evaluate the progress. How do we measure our goal of creating safe systems inside health care organizations and—even more specifically—creating safe practices at the clinical interface to prevent WSP?

One method of evaluating WSP is to learn from the error and prevent future risk, which can be done by investigating the root cause or the basic reason for the failure of the process through a root cause analysis. Dattilo and Constantino[36] defined a root cause analysis as "the process of learning from consequences wherein health care providers take a step back and gain knowledge from near-misses, adverse events, or sentinel events in the operating room and all areas of health care." A WSP root cause analysis should include all participants who are directly or indirectly involved in the procedure: surgeons, nurses, surgical technologists, anesthesia providers, managers, directors, vice presidents, risk managers, and safety officers. Even the patient and family perspective can reveal contributing factors. Administrator participation is important because these leaders have the authority to change systems and the environment to support necessary improvements in the action plan.

The perspective and perceptions of all players heighten the illumination of multiple processes and factors frequently occurring in parallel that impact on disruption of the patient care process, which can potentially result in a WSP. Results of the root cause analysis often do not find just one reason or breakdown that caused the WSP. The process involves using fishbone diagrams to map out the causes and effects related to the WSP. The Joint Commission developed a root cause analysis matrix to map out areas of inquiry for specific sentinel events. Minimally, they require the following processes to be included in a root cause analysis of a WSP: physical assessment, patient identification, staffing levels, orientation and training of staff, competency assessment/credentialing, communication with patient/family, communication among staff members, availability of information, and physical environment.[37] For each area of discovery, an action plan is developed, the responsible party is identified, and implementation time frames are set. The outcome must be to reduce or eliminate the risk to patients in the future, and the mode of measuring this is elimination of WSP.

Universal reporting of medical errors and near misses is another suggested method of measuring improvement in WSP. It is expected that the system meet three basic principles: anonymity, nondiscovery, and nonpunitive. Numerous reporting systems have been implemented throughout private and public establishments across the United States with the purpose of monitoring and evaluating the quality of health care. Andrus and colleagues[38] discussed many of the barriers to implementing such a program. "Error-reporter buy in" heads their list, because they believe "the completeness of any error-reporting process is directly proportional to all the critical elements of anonymity, nondiscoverability, a nonpunitive process and an individual's personal risk." Eliminating the risk is accomplished through a fourth principle of immunity for the committer and reporter of the errors. This principled process also would negate the ability of a patient's right to take legal action, a definite barrier. The authors see this as a practical solution to eliminate all disincentives to report and remind us that "error reporting should not be our goal, but only a means of learning from our short comings to help improve the future care of our patients."

There is a need for an enterprise-wide policy or procedure with the explicitly defined processes to meet the criteria in the Universal Protocol. Three things can be measured in relation to policy or procedure: whether one exists, staff knowledge of the policy or procedure, and whether it is being followed accordingly. Existence of the policy should be easy to evaluate, but one may want to examine the content to be sure it includes all aspects of the Universal Protocol criteria to prevent WSP and whether the criteria are being used. When assessing use of the policy, direct observation ensures validity and measures the use and practitioner knowledge. Medical record review can be done,

but that is retrospective and only substantiates documentation, not necessarily practitioner knowledge, communication methods, or performance of the policy content. Direct observation provides the opportunity to identify risks introduced by the policy and revise the policy based on provider feedback. Design of the measurement tool should evaluate practitioner behaviors, knowledge, and provide feedback.[19]

The Pennsylvania Patient Safety Reporting System demonstrated decreased frequency of wrong site surgeries. This is a mandatory reporting structure for all hospitals in Pennsylvania to report wrong site surgeries and near misses. In 2007, the Pennsylvania Patient Safety Reporting System conducted an observation of site verification processes at six Pennsylvania facilities. The goal was to understand the variations in interpretation and implementation of the Universal Protocol and how they might relate to WSP. One or more steps were observed for 48 procedures. Significant variation in implementation of the Universal Protocol and verification of information, site marking, and time-out procedures were noted. Noteworthy variations existed in all areas of the operative patients' journeys. In these observations and in a previous retrospective analysis,[15] the wrong site errors related to misinformation, which usually occurred preoperatively, or misperception, which occurred most frequently intraoperatively. In the retrospective study, incorrect information in preoperative documentation for surgery, schedule, consent, history, and physical resulted in 25 wrong site procedures out of 155 reviewed; misperception and right/left confusion resulted in 45 wrong site procedures.

The observation study allowed for real-time information gathering. Breakdowns were noted with incorrect consents when secondhand information was used and when verification of patient information was completed with passive acknowledgments. Errors were noted when marking the site did not involve patients or the mark was not consistent with all documents. Other issues developed when patients were turned to a position that resulted in left/right confusion and when regional blocks when performed before a time out was done. A correlation was found between attention in checking inconsistencies in documents and finding wrong site errors before the start of the procedure. The more frequently independent checks were performed, the less opportunity there was for misinformation to reach the OR and potentially harm the patient.[30]

Pronovost and colleagues[39] focused on the fact that health care lacks a structured approach to evaluation of the progress made in reducing the risk of events that cannot be measured in rates. WSPs are one of these risk events. Measurement is an absolute necessity if we are to evaluate improvement. It remains one of the challenges in addressing the problem of WSPs because practitioners and organizations may conduct an internal in-depth evaluation and root cause analysis of the "never events," but the results frequently remain private for fear of liability or media attention.[40] Without a reliable national database, understanding the scope of the problem of WSP is impossible. Without a culture of safety in which practitioners are provided a trusting environment with supportive processes for provision of patient care, the confidence in the team that anyone can stop the process if there is a question of safety, and a "just" response to error, we will not eliminate WSPs.

SUMMARY

Wrong site, wrong person, wrong procedure errors are preventable. Historical dealings with these mistakes frequently meant a search for the person to blame and shame. Current methodology demonstrates that often a break in the process or system has caused the error—not the people involved. This article examined initiatives that professional associations and regulatory, private, and public institutions are putting into place to prevent events that should never happen to patients, practitioners, or facilities.

REFERENCES

1. Canadian Orthopedic Association Committee on Practice and Economics. Position paper on wrong-sided surgery in orthopedics. Winnipeg, Manitoba, Canada: Canadian Orthopedic Association; 1994.
2. Canale TS. Wrong site surgery a preventable complication. Clin Orthop Relat Res 2005;433:26.
3. American Academy of Orthopedic Surgeons. Advisory statement on wrong-site surgery. Available at: www.aaos.org. Accessed April 27, 2008.
4. Joint Commission International Center for Patient Safety. Sentinel events alerts. Issue 6. Lessons learned: wrong site surgery. Available at: www.jcipatientsafety.org/14791/. Accessed May 8, 2008.
5. Kohn LT, Corrigan JM, Donaldson MS. To err is human building a safer health system. Washington, DC: National Academy Press; 2000.
6. Gaba D, Howard SK, Fish K. Crisis management in anesthesiology. NY (NY): Churchill-Livingston; 1994.
7. Brennan TA, Leape L, Laird NM, et al. Incidence of adverse events and negligence in hospitalized patients: results of the Harvard medical practice study I. N Engl J Med 1991;324:370–6.
8. Wong D, Mayer T, Watters W, et al. Prevention of wrong site surgery: sign, mark and x-ray (SMaX). LaGrange, IL: North American Spine Society; 2001. Available at: www.spine.org/smax.cfm. Accessed April 27, 2008.
9. Committee on Quality of Health Care in America Institute of Medicine. Crossing the quality chasm a new health system for the 21st century. Washington, DC: National Academy Press; p. 5–6.
10. Association of Registered periOperative Nurses (AORN). Correct site surgery tool kit building a safer tomorrow. Available at: www.aorn.org. Accessed April 25, 2008.
11. Joint Commission International Center for Patient Safety. International patient safety goals created. Available at: www.jcipatientsafety.org/show.asp?durki=11753. Accessed April 8, 2008.
12. Council on Surgical and Perioperative Safety. CSPS core principles. Available at: www.cspsteam.org/education2.html. Accessed May 14, 2008.
13. World Health Organization. Safe surgery saves lives initiative. Available at: www.who.int/patientsafety/challenge/safe.surgery/en/index.html. Accessed May 7, 2008.
14. The Joint Commission. Performance of correct procedure at correct body site. Patient Safety Solutions 2007;1(4). Available at: www.thejointcommission.org. Accessed May 12, 2008.
15. Clarke JR, Johnston J, Finley ED. Getting surgery right. Ann Surg 2007;246(3):397.
16. Manuel BM, Nora PF. Surgical patient safety essential is information for surgeons in today's environment. Chicago, IL: American College of Surgeons; 2004. p. 112.
17. Seiden SC, Barach P. Wrong-side/wrong-procedure, and wrong-patient adverse events: are they preventable? Arch Surg 2006;141:931–9.
18. Cowell HR. Wrong-site surgery. J Bone Joint Surg Am 1998;80:463.
19. Michaels RK, Makary MA, Yasser D, et al. Achieving the national quality forum's "never events" prevention of wrong site, wrong procedure, and wrong patient operations. Ann Surg 2007;245(4):526–32.
20. Joint Commission on Accreditation of Health Care Organizations. Sentinel event alert: a follow-up review of wrong site surgery. Report no. 24. Available at: www.thejointcommission.org. Accessed May 17, 2008.
21. Meinberg RG, Stern PJ. Incidence of wrong-site surgery among hand surgeons. J Bone Joint Surg Am 2003;85:193–7.
22. Understanding patient safety: a Q&A with Robert Wachter, MD. Infection Control Today 2008;3:54.
23. Kwan MR, Studdert DM, Zinner MJ, et al. Incidence, patterns, and prevention of wrong-site surgery. Arch Surg 2006;141:353–8.

24. The Joint Commission. Compliance strategies for the universal protocol. Chicago, IL: Joint Commission Resources; 2007. p. 11–7.

25. The Joint Commission, Joint Commission International, World Health organization. Performance of correct procedure at correct body site. Patient Safety Solutions 2007;1(4).

26. Cronen G, Vytantas R, Sogle G. Sterility of surgical site marking. J Bone Joint Surg Am 2005;87(10): 2193–5.

27. Norton E. Implementing the universal protocol hospital-wide. AORN J 2007;85(6):1187–97.

28. Bennett C. Timeout: it's easy as apple pie! OR Manager 2007;23(7):14.

29. Hylka SC. Ensuring consistent time-out in a system. OR Manager 2006;22(7):10.

30. Insights into preventing wrong-site surgery. Available at: www.psa.state.pa.us. Accessed May 14, 2008.

31. Landmesser S. A time-out tool helps improve compliance at the patient's bedside. OR Manager 2007;23(12):5.

32. Charlton N. Time out: the surgical pause that counts. AORN J 2004;80(6):1121–2.

33. Bloomfield C. Scripting for success. AORN J 2006; 83(5):1127–8.

34. Page L. System marks new methods of preventing wrong-site surgery. Mater Manag Health Care 2006;55–6.

35. Tablac A. Doctor's invention aims to prevent surgical mishaps. Available at: www.stltoday.com. Accessed November 5, 2007.

36. Dattilo E, Constantino RE. Root cause analysis and nursing management responsibilities in wrong-site surgery. Dimens Crit Care Nurs 2006;25(5):221–5.

37. The Joint Commission. Root cause analysis matrix minimum scope of root cause analysis for specific types of sentinel events: October 2005. Available at: www.jointcommission.org. Accessed June 1, 2008.

38. Andrus CH, Villasenor EG, Kettelle JB, et al. To err is human: uniformly reporting medical errors and near misses, a naive, costly, and misdirected goal. J Am Coll Surg 2003;196(6):914.

39. Pronovost PJ, Miller MR, Wachter RM. Tracking progress in patient safety: an elusive target. JAMA 2006;296:696–9.

40. Provonost PJ, Holzmueller CG, Martinez E, et al. A practical tool to learn from defects in patient care. Jt Comm J Qual Saf 2006;32:102–8.

To Count or Not to Count: A Surgical Misadventure

Cecil A. King, MS, RN, CNOR

KEYWORDS

- Surgery • Counts • Retained foreign body
- Recommended practices

On August 1, 2007, in the Inpatient Prospective Payment System Fiscal Year 2008 Final Rule, the Centers for Medicare and Medicaid Services[1] identified eight hospital-acquired conditions that are: (1) high cost or high volume or both, (2) result in the assignment of a case to a diagnosis-related group that has a higher payment when present as a secondary diagnosis, and (3) could reasonably have been prevented through the application of evidence–based guidelines. The first item on that list is a foreign object retained after surgery. For discharges occurring on or after October 1, 2008, hospitals will not receive additional payment for cases in which one of the selected conditions was not present on admission. That is, the case will be paid as though the secondary diagnosis were not present. What this means is that an unintended retained foreign body (RFB) has become one of the "never events" in an age in which both quality and efficiency are paramount and becoming more and more linked to pay-for-performance.[2] This then begs the question as to whether or not the Association of periOperative Registered Nurses' (AORN) *Recommended practices for sponge, sharps,* and *instrument counts* can be considered an evidence-based guideline. Would the routine counting of surgical instruments have prevented leaving behind a 2 by 13 inch malleable retractor? How does one explain this error to the patient, their family, and the public when something this large and obvious is left behind (**Fig. 1**)?

What happened in this case that predisposed it to an RFB? Two major patient safety issues became apparent during an internal claims closed-case review. One was the normalization of deviance, whereby there was a drift from the norm to the point that the deviance became the norm.[3,4] People cut corners and drifted from the norm (eg, counting of instruments) because until then nothing bad had happened. It was not the policy nor was there a procedure in place at this facility for the counting of instruments.[2] There was a generalized perception that instruments had never been left in patients at this facility, therefore the counting of instruments was not necessary. James Reason writes that, "All errors involve some kind of deviation. In cases of slips, lapses, and fumbles, actions deviate from the current intention."[5]

There is a growing body of evidence demonstrating risk factors related to RFBs. Gawande and colleagues,[6] in an analysis of errors reported by surgeons at three teaching hospitals, found that one-half to three-thirds of adverse events are attributable to surgery and that more than fifty percent are preventable. The incidence of RFBs has been reported somewhere between 1 in 9000 and 1 in 19,000 surgical cases (ie, .0001 to .00005), which may be translated to one or more a year within a large medical facility.[7] Greenberg and colleagues[8] reported that a discrepancy may occur in about one out of eight general surgery cases; with these discrepancies increasing the risk of an RFB. Given the risk and consequences related to RFBs and the fact that AORN's[9] *Recommended practices* represent "…what is believed to be an optimal level of practice (ie, care)," the perioperative nurse has a professional duty and an inherent ethical and legal obligation to prevent harm such as an RFB.

Cape Cod Hospital, 27 Park Street, Hyannis, MA 02601, USA
E-mail address: cking@capecodhealth.org

Perioperative Nursing Clinics 3 (2008) 395–400
doi:10.1016/j.cpen.2008.08.002

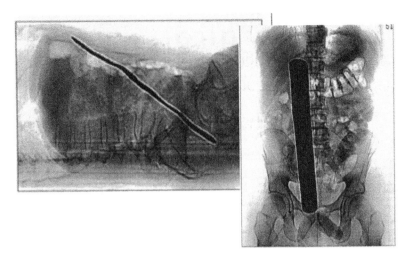

Fig. 1. Retained malleable retractor, 2001.

The law requires only that unintentional foreign bodies not be negligently left in patients. "The law does not prescribe how counts should be performed, who should perform them, or even that that they need to be preformed."[9] It is the individual perioperative nurse's professional responsibility to act as a prudent nurse would under the same or similar circumstances. It would behoove the prudent perioperative nurse to seek direction from AORN's *Recommended practices*[9] which recommends that sponges, needles, instruments, and other items "...be counted on all procedures in which the possibility exists that [an item] could be retained." The employer is responsible for the employee's actions that are taken within the scope of their employment. Upon accepting employment, there is an implied agreement between the perioperative nurse and the employer that she or he will perform within the standard of care (ie, standards of practice). The legal standard of care refers to what any prudent nurse with similar training, experience, or education would do in the same or similar situation. Failure to demonstrate this standard of care is considered negligence. The doctrine of *res ipsa loquitur* (ie, this thing speaks for itself) applies to RFBs, rendering this sort of litigation almost indefensible.[10] In cases involving an RFB, the retained object presents as prima facie evidence of negligence. Before 1977, the surgeon may have been held ultimately responsible for an RFB under the captain-of-the-ship doctrine. However, in 1977, the Texas Supreme Court ruled in favor of the surgeon, Sparger v Worley Hospital, Inc., 547 S.W. 2d 582 (Tex. 1977), refusing to apply the captain-of-the-ship doctrine by finding that the incorrect sponge count was the responsibility of the nursing staff, and, therefore the hospital.[11] Such a breach in one's

duty to deliver the standard of care or the failure to act as a reasonable person would act in a similar situation falls in the category of an unintentional tort or negligence.[10] While AORN is not a regulatory body, and therefore AORN's *Recommended practices* are not enforceable under the law, one's individual behavior is held up to that of the *Recommended Practices* since they are often cited as what a prudent nurse would do in the same or similar situation. Dr. Schroeter[12] describes the perioperative nurse's ethical obligation as it relates to practice standards by stating, "Nurses must be able to act to ensure that safe, competent, legal, and ethical care is provided to all patients."

Kaiser and colleagues[13] studied the frequency of occurrence of retained surgical sponges by examining RFB insurance claims over a seven-year period. Forty-eight percent (n = 40) of this sample involved retained surgical sponges. A falsely correct sponge count was documented in 76% of the abdominal cases in this study. In 1996, the costs were reported at $2,072,319 in total indemnity payments and $572,079 in defense costs. In 3 of the 40 cases, the surgeon was found guilty of negligence by the court despite the nursing staffs' admitted liability. In a retrospective study of 24 patients presenting with an RFB after abdominal surgery, Gonzalez-Ojeda and colleagues[14] reported that RFBs may occur at a rate of 1 in 1000 to 1500 open-abdominal procedures.

While there are upwards of 1300 published papers found when using the search terms "retained foreign body, surgery" at the PubMed Web site, the first comprehensive study to identify risk factors for RFBs was undertaken between 1985 and 2001. It used a retrospective case-control methodology of reviewing the medical records associated with claims and incidence reports of

RFBs. Gawande and colleagues[7] concluded that the risk of an RFB significantly increases during emergencies procedures, when there are unplanned changes in the procedure, and in patients with a significantly higher body mass index. In patients presenting with an RFB, it was less likely that a surgical count had been performed. Gawande and colleagues recommended that using a counting process similar to AORN's *Recommended practices*, monitoring personnel's compliance with the process, and using radiologic screening of patients at high risk for RFBs are measures that may be implemented to prevent an RFB. Based upon Gawande and colleagues' projections, the ratio of the number of radiographs it would take to detect an RFB is about 300 to 1, and very dependent on the quality of the film and expertise of the person reading the film. Yet the cost–benefit ratio is about $50,000 paid out in claims versus about $100 for the cost to obtain a plain radiograph to detect an RFB. Given the risk–benefit ratio to the patient, performing a plain radiograph to detect or rule out an RFB would seem a far more prudent practice than to do nothing at all.

So, what happened in the case depicted in **Fig. 1** that contributed to leaving behind a malleable retractor? The superseding casual effect was the normalization of deviance, a cultural-sociologic phenomenon whereby individuals or teams repeatedly accept lower standards of performance until the lower standard becomes the norm. There was a prevailing attitude of complacency about counting instruments because "nothing has happened so far." We see this often in health care, and eventually, the attitude that nothing has happened "yet" becomes the norm and therein lies the danger.[4] The facility in which this event occurred did not routinely count surgical instruments because "nothing has happened" and because the prevailing belief was that there was no data supporting the manual counting of instruments as a reliable method of prevention. "This again appears to substantiate the danger of not knowing what one does not know."[15] What was lacking was transparency and two-way communication between the risk management and claims departments, and the management of the operating room (OR). What would become evident upon closer examination was that there was indeed a problem; the incidence of RFBs averaged about 1.8 per year at this facility.

A benchmark survey of the area hospitals and members of the University Hospital Consortium (UHC) was conducted to assess the community standard related to the counting of surgical instruments. This e-mailed survey has no scientific rigor,

reliability, or validity and therefore should not be considered as evidence-based data. UHC was chosen as the comparative national benchmark as the event occurred at a major academic medical center and the investigator had access to the UHC perioperative staff e-mail directory. Of the 13 hospitals contacted within the urban area in which the incident occurred, 62% (8/13) counted instruments in cases as recommended by AORN. A much higher percentage, 95% (20/21) of academic medical centers responding to the survey reported counting instruments as outlined in AORN's *Recommended practices*. The largest response, 34, came from surveying AORN Member-Talk, an electronic interactive bulletin board. This indicated that of the 34 members responding 82% (28/34) reported counting instruments according to AORN's *Recommended practices*. It was apparent that the community standard at both the local and national levels was to count instruments as outlined in the AORN's *Recommended practices*.

The case received local and national media attention. The story, which focused on medical errors, and the patient's radiographs (**Fig. 1**) were published in the *New York Times*, and the patient appeared on the television program Good Morning America. It was discovered that, over the course of five years, the facility had experienced nine RFBs at a rate of 1.8 per year. A comprehensive evaluation of these cases was undertaken. **Box 1** lists the commonalities identified in a closed-claims review of these cases.

Box 1
Commonalities of RFBs in nine cases over five years
Surgical services
4 Cardiothoracic
3 Gynecologic
2 General surgery
Cavity of involvement
Thoracic or abdominal
Other factors
6/9 Involved a retained instrument
5/9 Incision was after 13:00
6/9 Cased finished after 15:00
7/9 Occurred on a Thursday or Friday
3 (on average) changes in nursing personnel between counts
n = 9 (1996–2001)
Incidence rate 1.8 year

The myth that "nothing had happened yet" was dispelled and work turned to focusing on eliminating barriers to performing instrument counts. The findings of the case-by-case analysis of the closed-claims cases was presented to a multidisciplinary quality improvement team who performed a root-cause analysis (RCA) of the case. The RCA identified the following factors as contributing to the RFB:

Inappropriate procedure (ie, not counting instruments on open-cavity procedures)
Potential for interruptions and distractions
Sets were too large with upwards of 250 or more instruments
Lack of experience or competence
Time of day
Variations in instrument tray set-ups
Variations in the process of counting
Transcription errors: circulator forgot to document items added or removed from the field
Lack of cooperation of the count process by the surgeons
Lack of consistency in assigning staff breaks and handoffs when going on break

Two immediate performance improvement (PI) activities were put into place. One was to work toward standardization and streamlining of instrument sets to facilitate the counting process. The second was to conduct a direct observation of the more common procedures to identify those instruments that were used consistently and those which were rarely used. This provided the team leaders with important data as they met with their respective surgeons and team members in working to reduce the number of instruments in any given set. The departmental patient safety initiative was that no patient was to leave the hospital with a retrained surgical instrument, sponge, or needle. Therefore, routine plain radiographs were obtained on all intracavity procedures while the instrument count process and education were being implemented. The following PI activities were put in place:

Identify procedures requiring instrument counts
Identify those sets needing reconfiguration
Reconfigure and reduce the number of instruments per set
Count instruments on all open-cavity procedures (eg, chest, abdomen, pelvis)
Revise surgical count procedure to reflect AORN's Recommended practices
Conduct demonstration and return-demonstration training and competency validation of counting process
Limit phone calls into the room
As they are scrubbed, surgeons (eg, residents) hand off pagers to covering colleagues
Implement one purposeful PI-risk management communication process
Develop an interdisciplinary PI process
Conduct a Failure Mode Effect Analysis of the count process

In spite of the data supporting the need to implement the manual counting of instruments, it was met with resistance by some of the nursing staff and surgeons who felt it would impede the flow of the case and jeopardize patient safety. Two very important lessons were learned. One was the impact on patient safety of normalization of deviance. The second was that without transparency and open communication between the leadership in the OR and risk management (eg, claims) there are missed opportunities for improvement because every miscount should be viewed as an opportunity for improvement. The danger lies in not knowing what you don't know.

Over the past five years, technological advances such as bar coding, electronic article surveillance and radiofrequency identification (RFID) have been applied to the problem of retained sponges. It is worth reiterating that most of these devices have focused on the detection of surgical sponges. Marcario and colleagues[16] reported 100% accuracy in the detection of tagged sponges using an RFID wand. Marcario and colleagues' findings should be considered with caution given the small sample size (n = 8) and given the limitation associated with the RFID wand. This clinical trial raised important user issues, not unlike the traditional manual counting method: there is always the chance for operator error and the user must know how to use the device correctly. For the scan to be done correctly it has to be performed no farther than a few inches away from the skin or the device will not read the entire area of the surgical site and a retained sponge may be missed. Retained sponges could also be missed if the scan is performed too early (eg, if additional sponges were placed in the wound during closure). An economic analysis of such a device is warranted to justify the additional cost of the device and tagged sponges. The average price for an RFID device runs about $144 per case, in addition to the added labor cost and time.

Greenberg and colleagues[18] conducted a randomized, controlled clinical trial to evaluate a computer-assisted method of counting bar coded sponges. The bar code method significantly increased the detection of misplaced and miscounted sponges. However, it is important to evaluate the effects of adjunct counting technology on workflow and personnel performance. Greenberg and colleagues reported that the introduction of the bar coding technology decreased perceived team performance and increased the time dedicated to the sponge count by about three minutes. However, by the end of the study, the majority of participants found the system easy to use, were confident in the system's ability to detect sponges, and reported an improvement in patient safety.

The emerging technological surgical count devices should be developed and investigated in such a manner as to evaluate both their statistical and clinical significance in light of their clinical practicality. Cost should be included in these evaluations and compared with the cost of a count discrepancy as reported by Egorova and colleagues.[19]

In January of 2008, two important studies were published in the *Annuals of Surgery*[19,20] that finally provided satisfactory evidence suggesting which approaches were more efficacious in the prevention of RFBs. These studies recommended both policy changes and further research as follows:

> The current manual counting process as outlined by AORN in the *Recommended practices for sponge*, *sharps*, and *instrument counts*[9] plays an important role in the detection of RFBs and should be used consistently. Egorova and colleagues are the first to publish the efficacy of manual counting and reported a sensitivity of 77% and a specificity of 99%. Only 1.6% of the discrepant counts were actually associated with RFBs.
>
> The potential for an RFB is increased 100-fold in the event of a discrepancy.[19]
>
> Any time there is a discrepancy in the manual count, a radiograph should be obtained unless the needle is less than 10 mm in size (ie, a suture of about 5-0 to 6-0).[20]
>
> The manual counting process can be detrimental in some circumstances.[21] Each facility should consider when it is in the best interest of the patient to abort the count (eg, life-threatening emergencies) and a radiograph should be performed routinely before the patient leaves the OR.[19]
>
> The routine use of a radiograph before the patient leaves the OR should be considered as an adjunct for all high-risk patients or during high-risk situations (eg, unplanned change in the procedure, emergency, bariatric patients).[7,17]

Further studies to look at the counting process to determine the rate at which discrepancies occur are warranted. While the projected incidence rates are low, they should be considered within the context that, for the most part, this information is obtained by voluntary reporting and there is a high probability that the incidence of RFBs is highly underestimated. The findings of Egorova and colleagues[19] suggest the incidence of RFBs is more common than previously thought.

An instrument or other surgical item left in the patient is a rare and yet devastating and preventable complication of surgery. Despite the increasing body of knowledge over the past decade, it has been difficult to quantify the frequency of this event and to validate that the manual counting process is an effective preventative method. The manual counting process has been shown to be labor intensive and to negatively affect the progress of the surgical procedure.[22] Until now there has been no data supporting the accuracy and reliability of manual counting. With the publication of Egorova and colleagues[19] and Ponrartana and colleagues[20] in the January 2008 issue of the *Annuals of Surgery*, we are able to better understand the utility of our current approach in the prevention of RFBs. What is needed to further advance any patient safety effort "…is a committed management team, inclusive of the chief executive officer and the board of directors, and a dedication to supervision, an educational program within which roles, responsibilities, and expectations are reinforced with all staff, including physicians. A thorough prevention, detection, and correction process must be aimed at eliminating risk but focused enough to detect and then communicate throughout the organization any correction interventions to assure prevention of a future event."[17]

REFERENCES

1. Centers for Medicare & Medicaid Services hospital-acquired conditions. Available at: http://www.cms.hhs.gov/HospitalAcqCond/06_Hospital-Acquired%20Conditions.asp#TopOfPage. Accessed June 29, 2008.

2. Thomas FG, Caldis T. Emerging issues of pay-for-performance in health care. Health Care Financ Rev 2007;29(1):1–4.

3. Marx D. Patient safety and the "Just Culture": a primer for health care executives. April 17, 2001. Available at: http://www.mers-tm.net/support/Marx_Primer.pdf. Accessed June 29, 2008.

4. Groom R. Normalization of deviance: rocket science 101. J Extra Corpor Technol 2006;38(3): 201–2.

5. Reason J. Safety in the operating theatre—part 2. Qual Safe Health Care 2005;14:57.

6. Gawande AA, et al. Analysis of errors reported by surgeons at three teaching hospitals. Surgery 2003;133(6):614–21.

7. Gawande AA, Studdert DM, Orav EJ, et al. Risk factors for retained instruments and sponges after surgery. N Engl J Med 2003;348(3):229–35.

8. Greenberg CC, Diaz-Flores R, Lipsitz S, et al. A prospective study of OR counting protocol. J Am Coll Surg 2007;205(3S):S73 [abstract].

9. AORN Recommended practices for sponge, sharps, and instrument counts. In: 2008 Ed. Perioperative standards and recommended practices. Denver: AORN; 2008. p. 293.

10. Aiken TD. Standards of care in. In: Bogart JB, editor. Legal nurse consulting principles and practice. Boca Raton (FL): CRC Press; 1998. p. 37–45.

11. Iyer PW, Aiken TD. Nursing malpractice. 2nd edition. Danvers (MA): Lawyers and Judges Publishing Company; 2001. p. 287.

12. Schroeter K. Unit 3-Patient advocacy. In: Ethics in perioperative nursing practice. Denver (CO): AORN; 2004. 24.

13. Kaiser CW, Friedman S, Spurling KP, et al. The retained surgical sponge. Ann Surg 1997;224(1): 79–84.

14. Gonzalez-Ojeda A, Rodriguez-Alcanar DA, Arenas-Marquez H, et al. Retained foreign bodies following intra-abdominal surgery. Hepatogastroenterology 1999;46(26):808–12.

15. Rhodes RS. Invited commentary: analyzing adverse medical events—it's the system. Surgery 2003; 133(6):625.

16. Marcario MD, Morris D, Morris S. Initial clinical evaluation of a handheld device for detecting retained surgical gauze sponges using radiofrequency identification technology. Arch Surg 2006;141:659–62.

17. Gibbs VC, Coakley FD, Reines HD. Preventable errors in the operating room: retained foreign bodies after surgery—part I. Current Problems in Surgery 2007;44(5):325–9.

18. Greenberg CC, Rafael D-F, Lipstiz SR, et al. Barcoding surgical sponges to improve safety: a randomized controlled trial. Annals of Surgery 2008;247(4)612–16.

19. Egorova NN, Moskowitz A, Gelijns A, et al. Managing the prevention of retained surgical instruments. What is the value of counting? Ann Surg 2008; 247(1):13–8.

20. Ponrartana S, Coakely FV, Yeh BM, et al. Accuracy of plain abdominal radiographs in the detection of retained surgical needles in the peritoneal cavity. Ann Surg 2008;247(1):8–12.

21. Dierks MM, Christian CK, Roth EM, et al. Healthcare safety: the impact of disabling "safety" protocols. IEEE SMC Transactions-part A: Systems and Humans 2005;34:693–8.

22. Christian CK, Gustafan ML, Roth EM, et al. A prospective study of patient safety in the operating room. Surgery 2006;139:159–73.

Index

Note: Page numbers of article titles are in **boldface** type.

Moving?

Make sure your subscription moves with you!

To notify us of your new address, find your **Clinics Account Number** (located on your mailing label above your name), and contact customer service at:

E-mail: elspcs@elsevier.com

800-654-2452 (subscribers in the U.S. & Canada)
314-453-7041 (subscribers outside of the U.S. & Canada)

Fax number: 314-523-5170

Elsevier Periodicals Customer Service
11830 Westline Industrial Drive
St. Louis, MO 63146

*To ensure uninterrupted delivery of your subscription, please notify us at least 4 weeks in advance of move.

ELSEVIER

United States Postal Service

Statement of Ownership, Management, and Circulation
(All Periodicals Publications Except Requestor Publications)

1. Publication Title
Perioperative Nursing Clinics

2. Publication Number 0 2 4 - 5 3 3 5

3. Filing Date 9/15/08

4. Issue Frequency
Mar, Jun, Sep, Dec

5. Number of Issues Published Annually
4

6. Annual Subscription Price
$107.00

7. Complete Mailing Address of Known Office of Publication (Not printer) (Street, city, county, state, and ZIP+4)
Elsevier Inc.
360 Park Avenue South
New York, NY 10010-1710

Contact Person
Stephen Bushing

Telephone (Include area code)
215-239-3688

8. Complete Mailing Address of Headquarters or General Business Office of Publisher (Not printer)
Elsevier Inc., 360 Park Avenue South, New York, NY 10010-1710

9. Full Names and Complete Mailing Addresses of Publisher, Editor, and Managing Editor (Do not leave blank)

Publisher (Name and complete mailing address)
John Schrefer, Elsevier, Inc., 1600 John F. Kennedy Blvd. Suite 1800, Philadelphia, PA 19103-2899

Editor (Name and complete mailing address)
Alexandra Gavenda, Elsevier, Inc., 1600 John F. Kennedy Blvd. Suite 1800, Philadelphia, PA 19103-2899

Managing Editor (Name and complete mailing address)
Catherine Bewick, Elsevier, Inc., 1600 John F. Kennedy Blvd. Suite 1800, Philadelphia, PA 19103-2899

10. Owner (Do not leave blank. If the publication is owned by a corporation, give the name and address of the corporation immediately followed by the names and addresses of all stockholders owning or holding 1 percent or more of the total amount of stock. If not owned by a corporation, give the names and addresses of the individual owners. If owned by a partnership or other unincorporated firm, give its name and address as well as those of each individual owner. If the publication is published by a nonprofit organization, give its name and address.)

Full Name	Complete Mailing Address
Wholly owned subsidiary of	4520 East-West Highway
Reed/Elsevier, US holdings	Bethesda, MD 20814

11. Known Bondholders, Mortgagees, and Other Security Holders Owning or Holding 1 Percent or More of Total Amount of Bonds, Mortgages, or Other Securities. If none, check box ☐ None

Full Name	Complete Mailing Address
N/A	

12. Tax Status (For completion by nonprofit organizations authorized to mail at nonprofit rates) (Check one)
The purpose, function, and nonprofit status of this organization and the exempt status for federal income tax purposes:
☐ Has Not Changed During Preceding 12 Months
☐ Has Changed During Preceding 12 Months (Publisher must submit explanation of change with this statement)

PS Form 3526, September 2006 (Instructions Page 1 of 3) (Instructions Page 3)) PSN 7530-01-000-9931 PRIVACY NOTICE: See our Privacy policy in www.usps.com

13. Publication Title
Perioperative Nursing Clinics

14. Issue Date for Circulation Data Below
September 2008

15. Extent and Nature of Circulation

		Average No. Copies Each Issue During Preceding 12 Months	No. Copies of Single Issue Published Nearest to Filing Date
a.	Total Number of Copies (Net press run)	700	700
b. Paid Circulation (By Mail and Outside the Mail)	(1) Mailed Outside-County Paid Subscriptions Stated on PS Form 3541. (Include paid distribution above nominal rate, advertiser's proof copies, and exchange copies)	213	184
	(2) Mailed In-County Paid Subscriptions Stated on PS Form 3541 (Include paid distribution above nominal rate, advertiser's proof copies, and exchange copies)		
	(3) Paid Distribution Outside the Mails Including Sales Through Dealers and Carriers, Street Vendors, Counter Sales, and Other Paid Distribution Outside USPS®	7	8
	(4) Paid Distribution by Other Classes Mailed Through the USPS (e.g. First-Class Mail®)		
c.	Total Paid Distribution (Sum of 15b (1), (2), (3), and (4)) ▲	220	192
d. Free or Nominal Rate Distribution (By Mail and Outside the Mail)	(1) Free or Nominal Rate Outside-County Copies Included on PS Form 3541	48	41
	(2) Free or Nominal Rate In-County Copies Included on PS Form 3541		
	(3) Free or Nominal Rate Copies Mailed at Other Classes Mailed Through the USPS (e.g. First-Class Mail)		
	(4) Free or Nominal Rate Distribution Outside the Mail (Carriers or other means)		
e.	Total Free or Nominal Rate Distribution (Sum of 15d (1), (2), (3) and (4)) ▲	48	41
f.	Total Distribution (Sum of 15c and 15e) ▲	268	233
g.	Copies not Distributed (See instructions to publishers #4 (page #3)) ▲	432	467
h.	Total (Sum of 15f and g) ▲	700	700
i.	Percent Paid (15c divided by 15f times 100)	82.09%	82.40%

16. Publication of Statement of Ownership
☑ If the publication is a general publication, publication of this statement is required. Will be printed in the December 2008 issue of this publication. ☐ Publication not required

17. Signature and Title of Editor, Publisher, Business Manager, or Owner _(signature)_ Finance – Executive Director of Subscription Services

Date September 15, 2008

I certify that all information furnished on this form is true and complete. I understand that anyone who furnishes false or misleading information on this form or who omits material or information requested on the form may be subject to criminal sanctions (including fines and imprisonment) and/or civil sanctions (including civil penalties).

PS Form 3526, September 2006 (Page 2 of 3)

Printed and bound by CPI Group (UK) Ltd, Croydon, CR0 4YY

03/10/2024

01040360-0012